CARDIAC RHYTHM DEVICES
A CASE-BASED APPROACH
TO MANAGEMENT

CARDIAC RHYTHM DEVICES
A CASE-BASED APPROACH
TO MANAGEMENT

Mehdi Razavi, MD
Director Clinical Arrhythmia Research
Texas Heart Institute
Assistant Clinical Professor of Medicine
Baylor College of Medicine
Houston, Texas

Alireza Nazeri, MD
Senior Cardiology Research Fellow
Texas Heart Institute
Houston, Texas

Ali Massumi, MD
Sultan Qabus Chair in Cardiac Electrophysiology
Director
Center for Cardiac Arrhythmias and Electrophysiology
Texas Heart Institute
Houston, Texas

Samuel J. Asirvatham, MD
Consultant
Division of Cardiovascular Diseases and Internal Medicine
Division of Pediatric Cardiology
Professor of Medicine
Mayo Clinic College of Medicine
Rochester, Minnesota

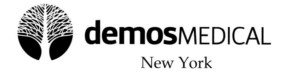

demosMEDICAL
New York

Acquisitions Editor: Richard Winters
Cover Design: Steve Pisano
Compositor: The Manila Typesetting Company
Printer: Hamilton Printing Company

Visit our website at www.demosmedpub.com

Medicine is an ever-changing science. Research and clinical experience are continually expanding our knowledge, in particular our understanding of proper treatment and drug therapy. The authors, editors, and publisher have made every effort to ensure that all information in this book is in accordance with the state of knowledge at the time of production of the book. Nevertheless, the authors, editors, and publisher are not responsible for errors or omissions or for any consequences from application of the information in this book and make no warranty, express or implied, with respect to the contents of the publication. Every reader should examine carefully the package inserts accompanying each drug and should carefully check whether the dosage schedules mentioned therein or the contraindications stated by the manufacturer differ from the statements made in this book. Such examination is particularly important with drugs that are either rarely used or have been newly released on the market.

Library of Congress Cataloging-in-Publication Data

Cardiac rhythm devices : a case-based approach to management / Mehdi Razavi ... [et al.].
    p. ; cm.
 Includes bibliographical references and index.
 ISBN 978-1-933864-67-9
 1. Cardiac pacing--Case studies. I. Razavi, Mehdi, M.D.
 [DNLM: 1. Pacemaker, Artificial--contraindications--Case Reports. 2. Arrhythmias, Cardiac--diagnosis--Case Reports. 3. Arrhythmias, Cardiac--therapy--Case Reports. 4. Cardiac Pacing, Artificial--Case Reports. WG 26 C2695 2011]
 RC684.P3C318 2011
 617.4'120645--dc22

                                                                                    2010024855

Special discounts on bulk quantities of Demos Medical Publishing books are available to corporations, professional associations, pharmaceutical companies, health care organizations, and other qualifying groups. For details, please contact:

Special Sales Department
Demos Medical Publishing
11 W. 42nd Street, 15th Floor
New York, NY 10036
Phone: 800–532–8663 or 212–683–0072
Fax: 212–941–7842
E-mail: rsantana@demosmedpub.com

Made in the United States of America
10 11 12   13   14   5 4 3 2 1

CONTENTS

FOREWORD

The field of medicine has gone beyond the longstanding prescribed require-ment of *Continuing Medical Education* as a method to maintain competence in a given field. We are now focused on 'life-long learning' in an effort to provide the best patient care in a discipline that is constantly changing and also for the purposes of credentialing and re-credentialing in our primary specialty, sub-specialties, and sub-sub-specialties.

Many would agree that there is no better way to maintain one's clinical skills and to prepare for credentialing and re-credentialing examinations than to work through 'real-world' cases.

Dr. Razavi and colleagues provide such real-world case examples in the discipline of implantable cardiac rhythm devices in this handbook. They have provided a broad selection of clinical cases that cover pacemakers, im-plantable cardioverter defibrillators, and cardiac resynchronization therapy devices. The reader has the ability to approach the case as an unknown as if they were seeing the patient, review the pertinent tracings and/or telem-etry, and decide on the best approach to management. This is followed by a discussion of the important clinical points that should be considered to optimize patient management.

This handbook will be helpful to any caregiver involved in the manage-ment of implantable cardiac rhythm devices for the purpose of providing improved patient care as well as for preparation of credentialing and re-cre-dentialing examinations.

David Hayes, MD
Division of Cardiovascular Diseases
Professor of Medicine
Mayo Clinic College of Medicine
Mayo Clinic
Rochester, Minnesota

PREFACE

The recent increase in utilization of implantable cardiac devices has made it ever more important for clinicians to have a fundamental understanding of this technology. While numerous comprehensive textbooks are available for an exhaustive study of the field, there remains a paucity of literature devoted to a detailed analysis of "real-life" intracardiac device tracings. We believe that the process of understanding the concepts represented in these tracings will enable the clinician to grasp the fundamentals underlying cardiac devices in an enjoyably challenging manner. This will enhance retention and comprehension of what is often and incorrectly thought of as an abstruse field.

Each of the tracings in this collection can be studied individually and in any order. For each tracing we have focused on the main interpretation in the hopes of discussing the most relevant clinical problem a clinician may encounter in the field It is our hope that after reading each case the readers will give themselves an opportunity to formulate a response before moving on to the discussion for the specific case. References are provided for those readers interested in a more in-depth review of the field.

This book is a quick reference for physicians and in-training house staff in the fields of cardiology as well as family medicine, internal medicine, and emergency medicine, and aims to assist in the diagnosis and management of common device-related clinical problems.

Mehdi Razavi, MD
Alireza Nazeri, MD
Ali Massumi, MD
Samuel J. Asirvatham, MD

Teaching Points

CARDIAC RHYTHM DEVICES
A CASE-BASED APPROACH
TO MANAGEMENT

PACEMAKERS

PACEMAKER TEACHING POINTS (PM)

CASE 1 Recurrent Syncope after Pacemaker Implantation

Case Presentation

A 53-year-old man underwent implantation of a dual-chamber permanent pacemaker 10 days ago for recurrent palpitations. The episodes were occurring on the average of once every 2 to 3 weeks and were associated with a prodrome of flushing and nausea. All of these occurred while he was working as a cashier in a supermarket. The physical examination, electrocardiogram, echo and stress test results had been normal.

A head upright tilt-table (HUT) test had been performed. The results demonstrated a sudden drop in heart rate 17 min into the study.

A diagnosis of neuorcardiogenic syncope with a predominant cardioinhibitory response was made. He underwent implantation of a dual-chamber pacemaker and was discharged without complication.

He now presents with two episodes of syncope in the last two days. They are associated with the same prodromes as previous. The prodromes last longer, and this gives him the chance to lay supine before loss of consciousness. The syncope itself lasted less than 10 s according to witnesses. Recovery was spontaneous.

The patient is asymptomatic at this time.

Examination is unremarkable except for mild orthostasis (supine blood pressure, 102/64 mm Hg; recumbent blood pressure, 94/58 mm Hg).

The supine rhythm and heart rate are sinus and 92 beats/min, respectively. Upon standing, however, it is noted that the patient's rhythm becomes paced as his heart rate drops to 60 beats/min. The rhythm is atrial paced with intrinsic ventricular conduction at rate of 120 beats/min.

Interrogation of the pacemaker demonstrates the following settings:

DDD, 50 to 130 beats/min
AV (sensed), 180 msec
AV delay (paced), 200 msec

The tracing is shown below (Figure 1):

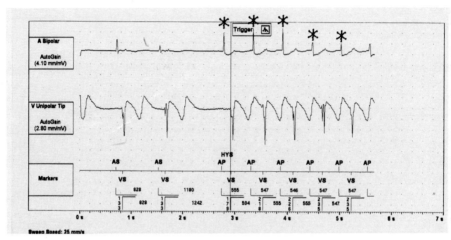

FIGURE 1

Case Discussion

Is the device working appropriately? Why was the rate response feature not turned on? Why did the patient have recurrent syncope?

Neurocardiogenic syncope (NCS) is defined as syncope caused by dysregulation of the autonomic nervous system. It is caused by inappropriate response to orthostatic challenge. It is manifested by a continuum between two extremes: *cardioinhibitory response* describes the condition wherein the primary response is a drop in heart rate induced by orthostasis, or other physiological stressors. *Vasodepressor response* is defined by a state of relative or absolute vasodilation in which vascular resistance, particularly of the venous capacitance vessels in the lower extremities, becomes impaired.

In both cases, the result is impaired central perfusion with secondary symptoms of light-headedness and syncope.

Most commonly, patients have a combination of these derangements, which may present with different extremes of each at different times. The underlying trigger, however, is usually orthostatic stress brought on by real or relative intravascular depletion. Thus, all patients with NCS should undergo conservative management in the form of aggressive hydration, use of lower extremity compression stockings, and sodium repletion if their blood pressure allows this.

In the current case, the results of the HUT demonstrated a drop in heart rate followed by syncope. Presumably, this cardioinhibitory response would be curable with a pacemaker. As noted above, however, patients may present with a combination or variety of response types in NCS.

The patient's history, physical examination, and investigations were suggestive of NCS: a "vagal" prodrome of nausea and flushing while in the recumbent position without evidence of structural heart disease. The presenting physiological abnormality cannot be reliably predicted by a HUT. Thus, despite placement of a pacemaker, attention still should be given to maintaining intravascular volume using the measures noted above. It may have even been reasonable to observe the patient's response to volume depletion before pacemaker implantation. Although studies have shown pacemakers to decrease the incidence of syncope, they cannot eliminate all such events.

The tracing demonstrates sinus rhythm with onset of pacing at 850 msec. This is shorter than the lower rate limit (LRL) of the pacemaker (1000 msec). The reason for this is that the pacemaker has a rate drop mode programmed on. In this case, the device is programmed to detect a sudden decrease in heart rate. This decrease is defined by the device and is programmable. The most common definitions incorporate the change in cycle length over a specified period of time.

In this example, the device was programmed to "detect" a drop in rate if there was a decrease of 20 beats/min over a maximum 30-s period. We can see onset of atrial pacing (star) at a higher rate once the "trigger" (vertical line) is declared. Thus, any decrease of 20 beats/min occurring over a period of less than 30 s triggered the feature. The response of the feature is also programmable but usually incorporates pacing at a higher rate for a period of time.

It should be noted that the heart rate need not drop below the lower rate limit of the device to declare a "rate drop" event. As such, pacing can occur at rate faster (or cycle length shorter) than the LRL, as seen in this case. The upper rate of pacing, however, does not violate the upper rate limit (URL). As such, the pacemaker demonstrated normal function.

CASE 2 Palpitations after Dual-chamber Pacemaker

TEACHING POINTS

- Pacemaker-mediated tachycardia
- Postventricular atrial refractory period
- Device malfunction

Case Presentation

A 62-year-old man is referred for ventricular tachycardia. He states that for the past two weeks he has been having frequent palpitations. Some of these last for minutes. The onset and termination are abrupt. There is no associated chest discomfort, shortness of breath, or light-headedness.

The episodes started two weeks after placement of a dual-chamber pacemaker. The pacemaker was placed because of symptomatic bradycardia.

He has no history of coronary artery disease or cardiomyopathy. His only medication is aspirin.

His examination is unremarkable. His resting electrocardiogram demonstrates sinus bradycardia.

You are asked to evaluate his rhythm.

Interrogation of his pacemaker shows no evidence of ventricular high rate episodes.

The device settings are as follows:

DDDR, 60 to 120 beats/min

Interrogation of his pacemaker during one of the episodes of wide complex tachycardia shows the tracing in Figure 1 on the following page.

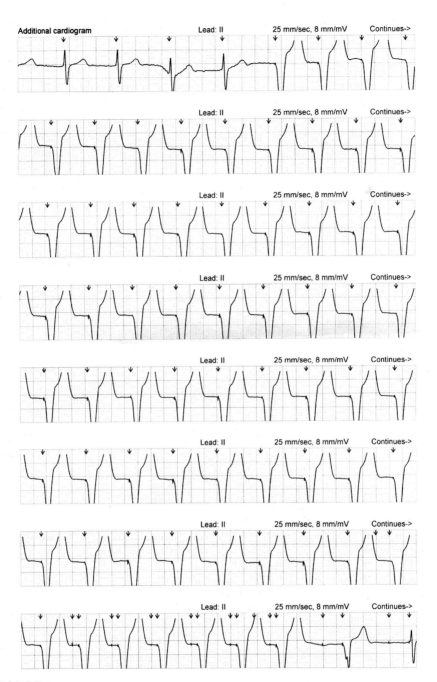

FIGURE 1

Case Discussion

Pacemaker-mediated tachycardia (PMT) is a form of endless loop tachycardia wherein an atrial sensed event leads to ventricular tracking (pacing). The ventricular impulse then travels in a retrograde direction, usually via the atrioventricular node, to the atrium. The atrial activation is then sensed by the atrial lead. This again leads to ventricular pacing, retrograde conduction of ventricular activation, and repetition of the circuit.

The common element in initiation of PMT is retrograde conduction of a ventricular impulse. The impulse can be due to ventricular pacing or intrinsic ventricular activation. A second requirement is presence of intrinsic ventriculo-atrial (VA) conduction. The VA conduction allows the atrial ventricular impulse to travel to the atrium. Once the atrial activation is sensed, ventricular tracking via the pacemaker follows (because the AV node will likely be refractory from the previous VA conduction). The ventricle is then paced. By this time, the AV node has recovered, once again allowing retrograde conduction and persistence of the tachycardia.

Thus, the most common clinical triggers for PMT are premature ventricular contractions, as they can lead to VA conduction, atrial sensing, ventricular tracking, and onset of tachycardia. Atrial undersensing can lead to PMT by leading to subsequent atrial pacing (without capture). Because the atrium does not capture, there is no AV conduction and ventricular tracking will ensue. The ventricular paced impulse can then conduct retrogradely to initiate PMT. Premature atrial contractions can be sensed, block in the AV node, and lead to ventricular pacing and initiation of PMT. To reiterate, any conduction associated with ventricular activation in the setting of an AV node that allows retrograde conduction is conducive for initiation of PMT.

In the tracing, sensed atrial events are followed by V-paced events (Figure 2 corresponds to the middle panels on the tracing in Figure 1). The atrial sensed events fall outside of the postventricular atrial refractory period (PVARP). Atrial sensed events falling within the PVARP are recognized but are not used to initiate an AV interval. Thus, ventricular tracking does not occur. This protects against the initiation of PMT. Extending the PVARP will increase the likelihood of the atrial sensed event falling within the PVARP and thus not being tracked.

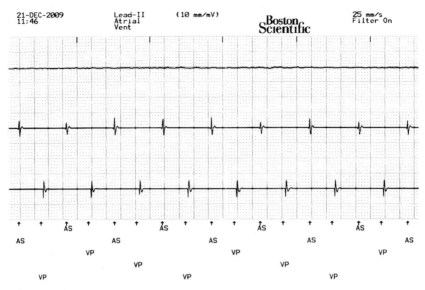

FIGURE 2

Placing a magnet on a pacemaker will eliminate all sensing. The pacemaker essentially starts pacing at the preset rate regardless of all external events. As noted, propagation of PMT depends on atrial sensing. Thus, when a magnet is placed on the pacemaker, the circuit is eliminated (atrial sensed event no longer leads to ventricular pacing). This terminates PMT and is indeed one of its diagnostic features. Atrial tachycardia with rapid tracking is not effected by a magnet.

CASE 3 A 72-year-old Man with a Pacemaker and Presyncope

TEACHING POINTS

- Upper rate behavior
- Pacemaker programmed intervals

Case Presentation

A 72-year-old man presents for routine pacemaker check. He received a dual-chamber pacemaker for severe AV nodal conduction disease. The device parameters are as follows:

DDDR's
LRL, 50 beats/min
URL, 130 beats/min
Sensed atrioventricular interval (AVI), 250 msec
Paced AVI, 270 msec
Postventricular atrial refractory period (PVARP), 330 msec

He informs you of recent onset of severe light-headedness brought on by vigorous exercise. This occurs during peak exercise, usually when his heart rate is in the range of 120 to 140 beats/min based on his wrist meter. He suddenly feels flushed and faint at the same time the monitor shows a rate of 50 to 70 beats/min.

He had not had any problems until recently when the β-blocker dose he was taking for the management of hypertension was decreased.

You decide to have the patient exercise on the treadmill.

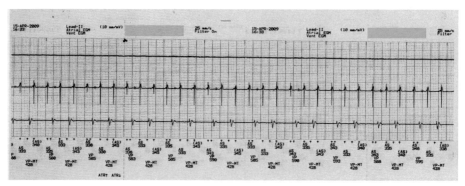

FIGURE 1

Case Discussion

What response do you expect to see as the sinus node accelerates? At what rate would this response be noted?

The upper rate behavior of a pacemaker is defined as the response to atrial sensed events in a patient whose AV conduction is dependent on the pacemaker.

Two responses are notable:

AV Wenckebach is a pattern in which the URL is achieved in the ventricle. In this scenario, the URL is reached in the ventricle because all atrial events are sensed (ie, are not in a refractory period). The relative frequency of nonconducted atrial events is a function of the ratio between these events and the URL of the pacemaker. Faster atrial events impose more frequent block of these events as the pacemaker cannot exceed the LRL. Wenckebach periodicity as defined by a shorter AV interval after the dropped beat than before the dropped beat is not observed, nor is progressive shortening of R-R intervals before a dropped beat.

A 2:1 AV block can abruptly occur if at a certain atrial rate, every other beat occurs during a refractory period. In this case, at a certain atrial cycle length, every other beat falls in the total atrial refractory period (TARP), defined as the combination of the AV interval and PVARP.

The clinical implication is important: once a patient's atrial cycle length (CL) becomes short enough so that every other beat is in the TARP, those beats fail to be sensed and tracked. This, in effect, leads to 2:1 AV block. The sudden drop in heart rate from the maximum tracking rate to one half that rate can be very symptomatic.

Shortening of the TARP requires short atrial CL (increased rates) for the onset of this phenomenon. This can be done by shortening either or both the AVI or PVARP.

There can be a transition from AV Wenckebach upper rate behavior to 2:1 block. This transition occurs when the atrial CL becomes shorter than TARP.

The rate at which this phenomenon occurs can be calculated by calculating the TARP. Thus, in this patient, TARP is 580 msec and 2:1 AV block would occur once the atrial cycle length shortens below this.

In this patient, very likely, withholding β-blockade enabled a higher sinus rate to be achieved. The cycle length shortened below TARP and symptomatic 2:1 block ensued.

The periodic nature of the ventricular paced rate may be explained by the fact that sensed P-waves close to the preceding paced QRS were in the post-ventricular refractory period.

CASE 4   A 52-year-old Man with Possible Pacemaker Malfunction and Syncope

Case Presentation

A 52-year-old man has a dual-chamber pacemaker. He presents to the emergency department with recurrent syncope. The episodes are not associated with any prodromes. He receives the pacemaker because of complete heart block.

His telemetry strip follows (Figure 1-A):

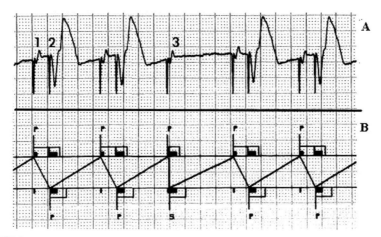

FIGURE 1

Case Discussion

What is the cause of the pacemaker's behavior?

The pacemaker is demonstrating the phenomenon of *crosstalk*. In crosstalk a paced atrial impulse in sensed in the ventricular chamber. Most frequently this occurs in pacemakers in the unipolar pacing mode. During unipolar pacing the vector of pacing is between the tip of the lead electrode and the pacemaker pulse generator ("can"). This leads to a wide area of electrical activity and increased propensity for sensing of the paced event in remote regions (such as the ventricle).

This causes the pacemaker to interpret the atrial *paced* event as a ventricular *sensed* event. If the pacemaker is programmed to inhibit pacing in response to a sensed event ("demand pacing"), the ventricular lead will respond by inhibiting pacing.

This can have catastrophic implications in a patient who is pacemaker dependent. Inhibition of ventricular pacing will lead to ventricular asystole.

It should be noted that the crosstalk, by definition, occurs only in response to ventricular sensing of a paced atrial event.

In the patient with delayed but intact AV nodal conduction, crosstalk is expected to lead to the observation of a prolonged paced AV interval beyond the programmed paced AV interval. This is because the paced atrial impulse has been sensed by the ventricular lead and has already led to the inhibition of ventricular pacing, or else ventricular pacing would have occurred at the end of the programmed paced AV interval. Intrinsic ventricular conduction is merely secondary (and very fortunate!).

In the current tracing Figures 1A and B represent AV sequential pacing and appropriate capture. The third atrial paced beat (3) demonstrated is not followed by a ventricular paced artifact. Figure 1B demonstrates why: the atrial paced impulse is sensed by the ventricular lead (note S [sensed event] on the bottom ventricular marker channel). The sensed event leads to the inhibition of pacing. Also of note, this sensed event (from atrial pacing) initiates a new VA interval that actually *pulls in* the next atrial paced event (P-P 880 msec, all beats but 800 msec from the nontracked atrial spike to the next atrial spike). Also keep in mind that AV conduction block makes these findings much more readily appreciated.

Management

The immediate management of crosstalk includes placement of a magnet that will revert the pacemaker to a "non-demand" pacing mode. No sensing or inhibition of pacing as a response to sensing will occur.

A ventricular *blanking period* is programmed and defines the period of time after an atrial paced (but not sensed) event during which the ventricular lead is refractory to sensing. In this situation, electrical after potentials from atrial pacing will presumably no longer be present, minimizing the risk of the ventricular lead sensing atrial pacing.

Programming to a bipolar pacing mode also minimizes the risk of crosstalk.

CASE 5 Device Management after Atrioventricular Node Ablation in an 82-year-old Man

TEACHING POINTS

- AV node ablation
- Sudden death
- Device troubleshooting

Case Presentation

An 82-year-old man has chronic atrial fibrillation with rapid ventricular conduction refractory to rate control medication.

A decision is made to proceed with AV nodal ablation and pacing.

After ablation of the AV node, the patient is left with an underlying heart rate of 30 beats/min and right bundle branch morphology.

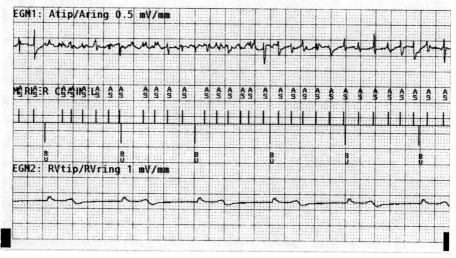

FIGURE 1

A biventricular pacemaker is implanted in the VVIR pacing mode.

Case Discussion

What specific precautions must be undertaken in the programming of the device?

What are the potential complications of this procedure?

Pacemaker implantation and AV nodal ablation leave most patients dependent on the pacemaker for cardiac activation. As such, any mechanical or other issues about integrity of the pacemaker can have catastrophic clinical consequences.

Until recently, there has been a small but real association between sudden death and AV node ablation plus pacing. Although it may seem intuitive that the underlying causes of death are issues regarding the integrity of the pacing system, more recent data have suggested that the mechanism of death is polymorphic ventricular tachycardia. The mechanism for the phenomenon is unknown, but speculation surrounds the sudden decrease in heart rate (recall most patients undergoing ablation have had rapid ventricular rates). It is thought that the decrease in rate alters the repolarization properties of the ventricle such that there is increased predisposition to such arrhythmias. Death frequently occurs weeks after AV nodal ablation.

It has been suggested that one means of eliminating the risk for polymorphic ventricular tachycardia is setting a relatively high lower rate limit for the pacemaker and gradually decreasing this setting. A common practice is to start at 80 or 90 beats/min and drop the lower rate by 10 beats/min on a monthly basis until a lower rate of 50 or 60 beats/min is achieved. Many individual practitioners have different approaches. Although controlled trials are lacking, anecdotal evidence suggests that this protocol can significantly decrease the incidence of sudden death after AV node ablation and pacing.

CASE 6　A 75-year-old Woman with a Pacemaker and Syncope during Prayer

TEACHING POINTS

- Lead fracture
- Device malfunction
- Oversensing

Case Presentation

A 75-year-old woman presents with syncope. She had a pacemaker implanted because of sick sinus syndrome and progressive AV nodal conduction system disease. The episodes of syncope have no prodromes and last a few seconds.

All episodes occur around 10 PM, as she prepares for bed. They are not associated with any changes in position. She does not take any diuretics or other blood pressure medications and denies positional light-headedness. A recent nuclear stress test showed normal left ventricular function without ischemia or scar.

Examination is unremarkable. Blood pressure measurements fail to demonstrate any orthostatic changes.

Electrocardiogram demonstrates sinus rhythm with a paced ventricular rhythm.

Her pacemaker is a dual-chamber pacemaker with the following settings:

DDDR, 50 to 120 beats/min
Sensed AVI, 180 msec
Paced AVI, 200 msec

Interrogation demonstrates normal sensing, pacing thresholds, and battery function.

The patient had an underlying ventricular rate of 30 beats/min.

Case Discussion

What other investigations are appropriate at this time?

Syncope in a patient with a pacemaker consists of the following differential diagnoses:

1. Vasodepressor response: unlikely given the history and physical examination findings.
2. Ventricular tachyarrhythmias: less likely given absence of anginal stress test, normal examination, and recent stress test.
3. Noncardiac causes: possible in this case. The absence of any prodromes or postictal symptoms renders this less likely.
4. Pacemaker malfunction: in a patient with known conduction system disease and syncope, bradycardia is the most likely cause of syncope. Detailed history is critical in elucidating a clear diagnosis.

Further questioning of the patient revealed that all episodes had occurred while she was praying before turning in at night. During prayer, she would sit on the floor and clasp her hands forcefully, pressing them against each other. She would lose consciousness a few seconds later.

What is the next appropriate step?

Anytime that physical motion of the arms or shoulders is associated with syncope in a patient with a pacemaker, there is concern for a mechanical problem leading to pacemaker malfunction. In such situations, it is best to interrogate the pacemaker while the patient is repeating the same physical activities. Even if the history is not specific, performing provocative maneuvers such as flexion/extension of the arms and shoulders or compression of the palms against each other can elicit the responsible mechanism.

In another case, during arm clasping, the following tracing was obtained:

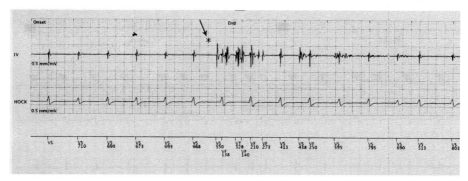

FIGURE 1

What does this tracing demonstrate?

The tracing demonstrates high-frequency ventricular sensed events during arm clasping (asterisk). The cycle length of these events is too short to be physiological and likely represents noise artifact. Given that these events were associated with mechanical maneuvers, they likely represent insulation failure or lead fracture. In both cases, noise is sensed as physiological activity and leads to inhibition of pacing. In the pacemaker-dependent patient, this leads to syncope.

CASE 7   A 54-year-old Man with Permanent Pacemaker Presents with Fever

---

TEACHING POINT

- Device infection

Case Presentation

A 54-year-old man with a history of heart failure and atrial fibrillation called the office complaining of fever and chills. He had undergone atrio-ventricular node ablation with pacemaker (PM) implantation 2 months prior. His cardiologist asked him to go to the emergency department. You were paged to see the patient.

Pertinent medical history and clinical presentation

He started having chills the day before admission. He also complained of pain and redness on his upper left chest on the area of the PM. He denied any other symptoms. His medical history included diabetes mellitus and myocardial infarction. He had coronary artery bypass surgery last year. His medications included insulin, atenolol, simvastatin, aspirin, enalapril, and warfarin.

On examination, he had a temperature of 100.4°F. The PM pocket was erythematous and tender to palpation but without fluctuation or signs of fluid collection. There was a 2/6 holosystolic murmur on the left sternal border and painful nodules on the second and third fingers of the left hand.

Case Discussion

Differential diagnosis

- PM pocket infection
- PM infection with endocarditis

Implantable cardiac device infection

Background:

- There are two main categories of device infections—(1) pocket infections: involve the subcutaneous pocket containing the device and the underlying leads but not the transvenous segment and (2) systemic infections: involve the transvenous portion of the lead, usually associated with bacteremia and/or endocarditis.

- Based on the source of infection, it can be classified as primary (the device or pocket is the source of infection) or secondary (the leads are seeded from another source). Device infection can be associated with valvular infection, although it may remain uninfected in the setting of valvular endocarditis. The true incidence of device infection is unknown but has been reported to be in the range of 0.8% to 5.7%. Several factors are associated with device infection: recent manipulation of the device (eg, generator exchange), previous temporary pacing, diabetes mellitus, malignancy, operator inexperience, older patient, treatment with anticoagulants or glucocorticoids, previous fever, and early reintervention.

Staphylococcus aureus and coagulase-negative staphylococci, often *Staphylococcus epidermidis*, cause more than two thirds of generator pocket infections and most device-related endocarditis. Infections within the first two weeks of implantation are mainly caused by *S aureus*. The most common organisms responsible for secondary infections is *S aureus* infections.

Streptococci, Corynebacterium species, Propionibacterium acnes, gram-negative bacilli, and *Candida* have been reported to cause pocket infections and device-related endocarditis.

Pocket infection commonly presents with fever and/or chills, general weakness, and other constitutional symptoms. Pocket infections can present with swelling, erythema, and pain at the site of the device in addition to systemic symptoms, particularly in the first few months after implantation.

Inflammation over the site or erosion of the device through the skin are highly consistent with pocket infection. The positive culture of material aspirated from the inflamed site confirms the diagnosis.

Transvenous electrode infection can effect intracardiac lead integrity and lead to right-sided endocarditis. Left-sided endocarditis is rare. The patient may present with sepsis syndrome and shock. The presentation is usually subacute. The common presenting symptoms are fever; chills; pulmonary involvement such as pneumonia, bronchitis, lung abscess, or embolism; tricuspid regurgitation; or mechanical stenosis from large vegetations. Epicardial electrode infection can present with signs of pericarditis or mediastinitis. Bacteremia is usually present.

Up to 50% of patients with device-related endocarditis have evidence of vegetation on a valve, most commonly the tricuspid valve. By adding the pertinent pocket abnormalities and pulmonary emboli as clinical variables to the major Duke criteria, a clinical diagnosis of device-related endocarditis can be made in most of the confirmed cases.

In the evaluation of patients with suspected device-related endocarditis and nondiagnostic transthoracic echocardiogram, information from a transesophageal echocardiogram should be used in the modified Duke criteria.

Initiation of empiric antistaphylococcal antibiotics in case of suspected pocket or generator infection is recommended. Considering the high incidence of methicillin resistance *S aureus* and *S epidermidis*, initial therapy with vancomycin is reasonable. In the case of device-related endocarditis or pocket infection with bacteremia, empiric antibiotic therapy of endocarditis is recommended. The antibiotic regimen can be changed once the causative organism(s) is (are) identified in blood and/or wound cultures.

In the current case, a transesophageal echocardiogram was ordered and revealed a vegetation on the right ventricular lead with no evidence of valvular endocarditis. The blood culture was positive for *S epidermidis*.

Critical management questions

Would you explant the device, lead, or both?
What is the duration of antibiotic therapy?

The device should be removed when there is pocket infection with or without associated bacteremia or lead infection, with or without endocarditis.

Device explanation is also recommended for patients with the following:

- *S aureus* bacteremia in the absence of an alternative source.
- Bacteremia that persists or recurs with no alternative source despite appropriate antibiotic therapy.

In the setting of infection limited to the pocket or subcutaneous tissue, it is recommended to continue antibiotics for 10 to 14 days after explantation of the infected system. The transition to oral antibiotics depends on the presence of systemic signs of infection, the local infection severity, and the urgency of implanting a new system.

When and where to implant the new device?

Until the initial infection is fully treated or controlled, reimplantation should not be attempted. In PM-dependent patients, temporary transvenous pacing should be continued until blood cultures are negative and endocardial infection has been controlled. This may require two weeks of parenteral therapy. However, in patients with pocket infections and no bacteremia or endocarditis, the new device can be implanted in a new location soon after explantation.

The new device should be implanted at a different site from the explanted infected system, ideally on the opposite side.

In the current case, after two weeks of therapy, the systemic symptoms resolved and repeat blood cultures were negative. The new PM was implanted and patient was discharged home on oral antibiotics.

Besides the routine PM care recommendations, is antibiotic prophylaxis recommended?

Transient bacteremia due to mucosal trauma rarely causes device infection. In the absence of another independent risk factor for endocarditis, antibiotic prophylaxis is not routinely recommended for patients with PMs or implantable cardioverter defibrillators. Some experts recommend antibiotic prophylaxis for procedures such as endoscopy, cystoscopy, or dental work in the first two months after implantation, before endothelialization is complete.

CASE 8   A 56-year-old Man with Possible Device Malfunction

TEACHING POINTS

- Ventricular safety pacing
- Crosstalk

- Oversensing
- Pacing inhibition

Case Presentation

A 56-year-old man with a dual-chamber pacemaker is noted to have the following rhythm strip shortly after aortic valve surgery (Figure 1).

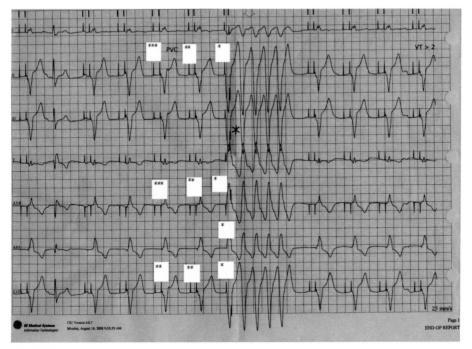

FIGURE 1

Case Discussion

What observation can you make regarding the pacemaker's behavior?

The first two beats demonstrate AV sequential pacing.

Subsequently, five beats of a regular wide complex tachycardia is noted. The tachycardia is not preceded by any P waves and thus represents ventricular tachycardia (VT). After termination of the VT, AV sequential pacing resumes.

Simultaneous with the onset of VT, the first of two pacing spikes are observed (asterisk). The first of the two spikes is exactly the same interval from the previous atrial spike (double asterisk) as the two previous atrial spikes were from each other (triple asterisk) (840 msec). This makes the first spike, simultaneous in onset with VT, likely an atrial spike. The following spike is therefore a ventricular pacing spike.

Shortly after the first spike, and at an interval of about 100 msec, the ventricular spike is noted (asterisk). This is considerably shorter than the previous intervals (160 msec).

This likely represents ventricular safety pacing (VSP). During VSP, if the ventricular lead senses any event within safety pacing interval, a ventricular pacing spike is delivered. The VSP is initiated shortly after every atrial pacing spike.

Its purpose is to prevent *crosstalk*. Crosstalk refers to inhibition of ventricular pacing due to sensing of the atrial pacing spike by the ventricular lead. In other words, the ventricular lead erroneously assumes that the sensed atrial spike is ventricular activity. In a patient with AV block, such inhibition would lead to asystole. To avoid this situation, the ventricular lead is programmed to deliver a rapid pacing spike after sensing *any* electrical activity after atrial pacing. Of two situations, one will be operative: if the sensed event was atrial in origin, the ventricular pacing is appropriate. If the sensed event was truly ventricular, the fact that the ventricular pacing occurred rapidly assures that the ventricular spike will not be proarrhythmic ("spike on T wave").

In the current tracing, the atrial spike leads to the initiation of a safety pacing interval on the part of the ventricular lead. Because of the simultaneous onset of VT, the ventricular lead senses activity immediately after atrial pacing (during safety pacing interval). The response will be VSP 80 msec later.

CASE 9　A 73-year-old Woman with Possible Pacemaker Noncapture

TEACHING POINTS

- Threshold testing
- Oversensing

- Noncapture

Case Presentation

The tracing below was obtained from the monitor in a 73-year-old woman who had undergone dual-chamber pacemaker implantation one day before (Figure 1).

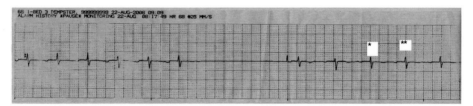

FIGURE 1

The device settings were as follows:
DDDR, 60 to 110 beats/min
Sensed AVI, 180 msec
Paced AVI, 200 msec

Case Discussion

Is there evidence of device malfunction? If so, which of the lead(s) is/are involved?

An initial review of the tracing shows what appears to be intrinsic P waves followed by a pause. Approximately 1.4 s later, an atrial pacing spike (asterisk) is observed. This appears to capture the atrium and conduct to the ventricle. This is then followed by P waves with intrinsic ventricular conduction.

The absence of pacing after the last P wave before the 1.4-s pause suggests oversensing and inhibition of pacing by the atrial lead. Similarly, the absence of ventricular pacing during the same interval suggests ventricular lead oversensing.

Also of note, the PR intervals after the pause (double asterisks) are longer than the programmed intervals, further suggesting ventricular oversensing, and pacing inhibition.

Thus, on initial review, it may be concluded that neither lead is functioning appropriately.

Closer inspection, however, demonstrates that the atrial rate after the pause is slower than that before the pause.

In fact, what occurred in this case was that pacemaker thresholds were being checked the morning after implantation. During assessment of atrial pacing thresholds, the pacemaker is temporarily set to atrial pacing without ventricular tracking (AAI). Atrial pacing spikes are not observed because their output is just above the capture threshold. During the pause, the output is subthresholded and not observable on the rhythm strip. Immediately thereafter, the atrial output is increased to maximum with a lower rate limit of 60. This leads to a visible pacing spike followed by atrial capture. There is subsequent onset of spontaneous atrial activity (note the rate is slower than that before the pause) with intrinsic conduction.

This more rapid rate of atrial pacing during threshold testing had led to overdrive suppression in this patient with severe sick sinus syndrome. Atrial noncapture with amplitude decrement (part of the automatic threshold test) manifested the sinus pause. A similar observation had been made during an electrophysiology study.

Take-home points are as follows:

1. Rhythm strips are not reliable markers of pacing spikes.
2. If it appears that there are multiple device malfunctions (in this case, oversensing of both atrial and ventricular leads), it is best first to investigate the scenarios under which the observations were made.

CASE 10 Multiple Pacing Artifacts in a Critically Ill Patient

---

TEACHING POINTS

- Device-device interactions
- Pacemaker-dependent patients
- Undersensing
- Noncapture

Case Presentation

The following tracing was obtained from a 69-year-old man in the intensive care unit (Figure 1). The patient has a history of atrial fibrillation and sick sinus syndrome for which he received a single-chamber atrial (AAIR) pacemaker.

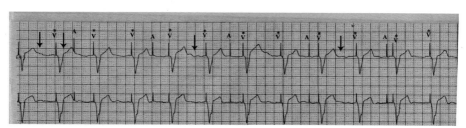

FIGURE 1

He is admitted with fevers, chills, and syncope. Blood cultures were positive for gram-positive cocci.

Case Discussion

What observations can be made?

Three immediate observations can be made: (1) the underlying rhythm appears to be either atrial flutter or fibrillation (arrows), (2) the ventricular rhythm is paced at a regular interval (V), and (3) two groups of pacing spikes can be observed (V for Vpace and A for Apace).

One of those spikes is the ventricular lead pacing at regular intervals (star). The other is the atrial lead, which does not appear to be capturing the atrium.

The atrial lead is pacing because it cannot sense the atrial fibrillation or flutter activity. However, it cannot capture the atrium because it is being constantly activated by the arrhythmia.

The ventricular lead is, in fact, a temporary pacemaker placed because the patient has bacterial endocarditis, which has destroyed the AV conduction system creating AV block and causing syncope. Thus, the patient has two independent pacing systems.

CASE 11   A 74-year-old Man with Dual-chamber Pacemaker and Shortness of Breath

Case Presentation

The following tracing was obtained from a 74-year-old man with a dual-chamber pacemaker (Figure 1).

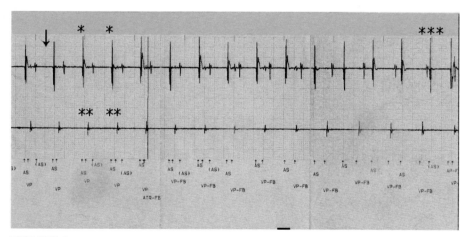

FIGURE 1

The patient had a history of atrial arrhythmias and sinus node dysfunction. He presented with onset of increased fatigue and shortness of breath.

Case Discussion

Based on review of the tracing (Figure 1), are there any observations that may explain the patient's symptoms?

Two channels are shown. The top channel is the atrial channel; the bottom is the ventricular channel. Below the channels are the electrogram markers, which represent the pacemaker's interpretation of the raw signals demonstrated on each channel.

The first beat demonstrates an atrial sensed (AS) event (star) followed by a ventricular paced event (VP) (double star).

Detailed attention to the atrial signals reveals that there is a signal after the first AS signal. This second signal is slightly later than the ventricular paced signal and reflects either far-field sensing of the ventricular event by the atrial lead or retrograde ventriculoatrial conduction via the AV node. Although the signal is seen in the atrial channel, we know that it is not interpreted as an atrial event because there is no corresponding marker on the marker channel.

The subsequent beats, however, demonstrate this second component to be interpreted by the pacemaker with the following marker: (AS). This universally can be interpreted as the pacemaker having sensed an atrial event but that it has chosen to ignore it because it is in a refractory period. The latter is demonstrated by surrounding the AS by parentheses. Although the device will "ignore" such AS events for the purpose of initiating an AV timing interval, it will not do so for the purposes of detecting (or "declaring") an atrial tachyarrhythmia.

As such, shortly after sensing the second atrial component on 3 successive beats, the device declares initiation of atrial arrhythmia (ATR-FB). The device then changes its pacing mode from a tracking mode (ventricular pacing in response to atrial sensing) to a nontracking mode wherein ventricular pacing is independent of AS events. This is referred to as *mode switching* and serves the purpose of avoiding rapid tracking of nonphysiological atrial arrhythmias.

It can be appreciated the after ATR-FB, ventricular pacing becomes independent of AS events. Detailed analysis of the penultimate (triple star) beat also clarifies the etiology of the second component of the atrial electrogram. Note that after mode switching, the second component is always preceded by ventricular pacing. This, as noted above, may indicate retrograde VA nodal conduction or far-field sensing by the atrial channel. In the penultimate beat, V pacing is followed by the atrial signal, which is immediately followed by an AS event. We know that two successive atrial events cannot occur so rapidly as atrial refractoriness is expected to occur. This then indicates that the second component is indeed far-field sensing of a true ventricular event by the atrial lead.

Finally, with regard to the patient's symptoms, it can be appreciated that once ATR-FB is declared, there is no further AV synchrony, as the pacemaker is in a nontracking mode. Although in reality, there are no atrial arrhythmias, the loss of AV synchrony can lead to loss of the physiological "atrial kick" and, in the case of this patient, multiple symptoms.

CASE 12 Ventricular Tachycardia in a Patient with a Dual-chamber Pacemaker

Case Presentation

A 62-year-old female with sick sinus syndrome underwent radiofrequency ablation of atrial fibrillation. She has a dual-chamber pacemaker. The morning after her procedure, you are called to assess a wide complex tachycardia noted on telemetry.

The tracing below is obtained (Figure 1):

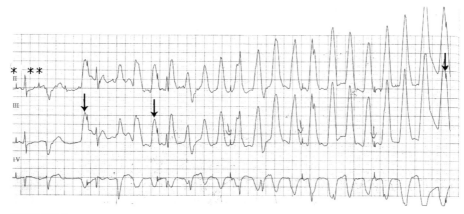

FIGURE 1

Case Discussion

What is the underlying rhythm?

Initial evaluation of the tracing demonstrated a wide complex tachycardia. This is concerning for ventricular tachycardia (VT). Closer inspection, however, demonstrates that the first impulse is an atrial paced beat with intrinsic ventricular conduction (star and double star). The atrial pacing artifact is followed by a captured P wave and intrinsic QRS. In the midst of the wide complex beats, these atrial impulses can be seen with regular frequency (arrows). This suggests that atrial pacing is occurring at a regular interval despite what, on initial glance, appears to be possible VT. Ventricular pacing is also possible but less likely as the morphology of the spikes looks consistent. Further analysis actually reveals what are most likely intrinsically conducted QRS complexes, which have been distorted. These also occur at regular intervals after each atrial paced beat, again making ventricular spikes less likely. These intervals approximate the spike-QRS interval of the first beat.

A pacemaker is very unlikely to continue atrial pacing during VT. One circumstance in which this could occur would be undersensing of VT. In that situation, however, one would expect to see ventricular pacing spikes. This is not seen in the current tracing. Even more suggestive against a diagnosis of VT are the discernible conducted QRS complexes.

Put together, these observations suggest that the wide complex tachycardia is likely an artifact.

Features that are suggestive of noise in a patient with a pacemaker and wide complex tachycardia are as follows:

- Absence of symptoms
- Regular pacing spikes or QRS morphology
- Source of ambient noise or interference
- History of Parkinson disease

The differential diagnosis of a wide complex tachycardia in patient with a pacemaker includes the following:

- VT
- Inappropriate ventricular pacing
- Artifact
- Supraventricular tachycardia (SVT) with aberrancy

Interrogation of the device confirmed the absence of any VT during the episode with consistent atrial pacing and intrinsic ventricular conduction.

Although ambient noise can create a high-frequency (often 60 Hz) artifact on telemetry leads, so can movement disorders such as Parkinson disease. Motion on the part of the patient can also lead to distortion of the signals. Surface lead movement or dislodgement can cause artifact but is unlikely in this case, as the intrinsic cardiac activity remained recorded during the course of artifact recording.

CASE 13 Ventricular Tachycardia Detected during Pacemaker Interrogation

TEACHING POINTS

- High-rate episodes
- Ventricular tachycardia
- Marker channel analysis

Case Presentation

You are informed by the pacemaker nurse that one of your patients has had multiple ventricular high-rate episodes detected on her pacemaker. The device is a dual-chamber Medtronic pacemaker and is programmed to detect ventricular high-rate episodes (VHREs) at a rate of 180 beats/min at 5 beats. The longest and fastest episodes' electrograms are stored.

The tracing below is representative (Figure 1):

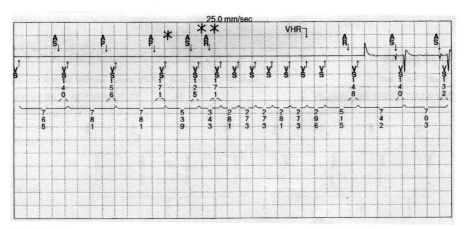

FIGURE 1

Case Discussion

What further evaluation may be considered? What is the most likely diagnosis?

The tracings show the atrial and ventricular channels. Analysis shows an abrupt increase in the ventricular rate. It is challenging, if not impossible, to assess changes in the ventricular morphology of the rapid beats. The atrial channel demonstrates a rate slower than the ventricle. This feature is suggestive of ventricular tachycardia (VT), and the pacemaker has accordingly placed this in the VHRE bin. There are, however, other causes for a V rate greater than A. These include junctional or atrioventricular nodal reentrant tachycardias with retrograde atrial block or ventricular channel noise.

Closer inspection demonstrates that at the onset of the VHRE, and immediately preceding it, one can observe atrial premature activity (star), which is followed by the first ventricular premature beat. Another atrial premature impulse can also be seen, followed by a train of ventricular beats. During the remaining course of the ventricular run, only one more atrial impulse is seen.

Once the VHRE is completed, atrial and ventricular sensed events (presumably sinus) follow.

One observation in this tracing is that the first premature beat is of atrial origin and is followed by a ventricular impulse. This may lead to the interpretation that the entire episode is of atrial origin. If this is the case, then one has to explain why there is no atrial sensed event for most of the VHRE. A number of explanations can be operative: first, if this was a brief run of atrial tachycardia (AT) with conduction to the ventricle, it may have led to atrial undersensing of the AT simply because these are of a different origin. The second explanation may be that the subsequent atrial beats were in atrial blanking or refractory periods. That is, each ventricular conducted beats led to subsequent atrial blanking period, which did not allow detection of atrial activity. If this were the case, however, we would have expected to seen AR, a marker for atrial events sensed in the refractory period. Except for the second premature atrial beat, we do not see any such electrograms. This argues against AT with refractory or blanked atrial signals. It is theoretically possible that all atrial events were in the blanking period, which is not sensed or annotated. The blanking period, however, was very short (50 msec in this case), making blanking of all atrial events (if this were an atrial arrhythmia with rapid ventricular conduction) unlikely.

The second premature atrial event may represent retrograde conduction of the first beat of VT (double star). In this case, the first atrial premature beat coincidentally preceded the onset of VT.

Also note that the first sinus beat after the tachycardia occurs at a relatively close coupling interval. If this were an AT, some degree of sinus node suppression would be expected after the termination of the tachycardia. This is not observed.

Another trick is to observe previous atrial high-rate episodes. If these are of the same rate as the VHRE, the conclusion that VHRE was of atrial origin is further supported.

Finally, and obviously, if electrograms were available, their review would have facilitated a diagnosis. In this pacemaker model, however, electrograms were not available.

The tracing is most likely demonstrating VT.

CASE 14 Intermittent Atrial Pacing in a 62-year-old Man with a Dual-chamber Pacemaker

TEACHING POINTS	
• Mode switching	• Atrial fibrillation
• Undersensing	• AV block

Case Presentation

The following ECG was obtained form a patient with a dual chamber pacemaker (DDD, 90 beats/min; AV interval 300 msec).

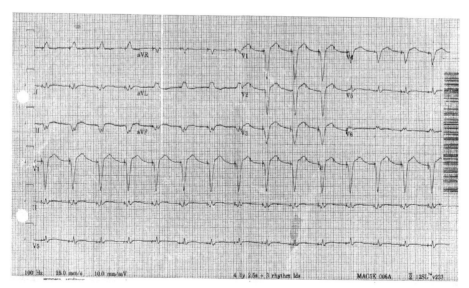

FIGURE 1

Case Discussion

What observations can be made?

The rhythm is ventricular paced at a rate of 90 beats/min. The first half of the electrocardiogram shows ventricular pacing. The second half demonstrates AV sequential pacing. The ventricular rate is unchanged.

Close inspection demonstrates the absence of P-waves throughout the tracing. Importantly, there appears to be no change in P-wave morphology, inasmuch as there is no discernable P wave with or without atrial pacing. When atrial pacing is present, the A-V interval is always timed out.

The patient is in atrial fibrillation (AF) with complete heart block. The first half of the tracing demonstrates sensing of AF by the atrial lead. The device goes into a mode switch (nontracking mode). In the second half, the atrial lead undersenses the fibrillatory atrial impulses and interprets the rhythm as atrial standstill.

Thus, atrial pacing commences. This obviously does not alter the atrial rhythm of AF. Because the patient has AV block, the AV interval times out. Ventricular pacing ensues.

This has no significant effect on the ventricular rhythm. Long-term consequences include premature depletion due to atrial pacing. The problem can be addressed by increasing the atrial lead sensitivity.

CASE 15   Tachycardia during Pacing

TEACHING POINTS	
• Cardiac arrhythmias in patients with pacemakers	• Pacemaker lead malfunction

Case Presentation

The rhythm strip on the next page was obtained from a patient with a dual-chamber (DDDR, 60–12) pacemaker.

Case Discussion

What observation can be made? What does this suggest about the nature of the tachycardia?

The rhythm strip initially demonstrates sinus rhythm with intrinsic AV conduction. There is appropriate sensing in the atrium and ventricle as manifested by the inhibition of pacing in both chambers.

Subsequently, an atrial pacing spike captures the atrium and conducts to the ventricle (arrow). We know that atrial capture occurs because the atrial spike leads to a premature P wave. The reason for the initiation of atrial pacing most likely is atrial undersensing, as the interval between the first atrial pacing spike and the preceding P wave is too short for the atrial lower rate interval to time out (intrinsic P wave to the next spike is a 620-msec [97 beats/min] interval). Subsequently, and at a regular interval of 1000 msec (the lower rate limit of the pacemaker), atrial pacing occurs. Some of these do not capture the atrium.

Before deciding if we are dealing with absence of atrial capture, it should be noted that intrinsic P waves have no effect on the atrial spikes. The P waves do not lead to atrial inhibition. Thus, one definite problem

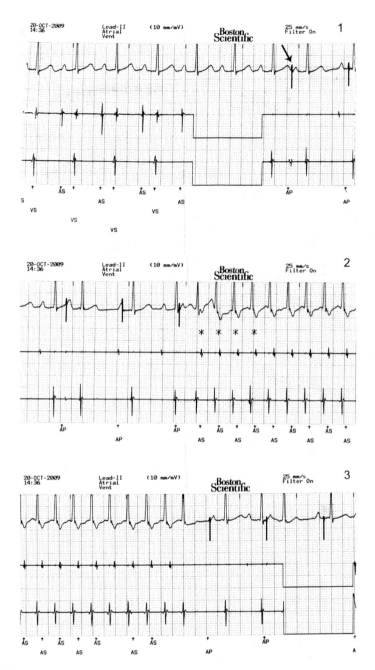

FIGURE 1

is atrial undersensing. Although it is true that the second atrial spike does not capture the atrium, it should be noted that a P wave immediately preceded it and that the atrium was likely refractory. The third spike does capture the atrium. The fourth spike occurs immediately after the P wave, and thus, the atrium was again refractory. The fifth spike, importantly, also captures the atrium. This is followed by a regular narrow complex tachycardia. Inverted P waves can be observed immediately after each QRS (asterisks). All ventricular pacing is inhibited.

The fifth atrial spike acted as a premature atrial contraction and led to the onset of a supraventricular tachycardia, likely AV nodal reentrant tachycardia. The absence of A pacing during the SVT suggests that the P waves during the tachycardia were sensed by the pacemaker.

Intermittent loss of atrial sensing eventually led to a captured atrial beat (fifth spike), which acted as a premature atrial impulse (PAC) to induce SVT. During SVT, the atrial electrograms were sensed with appropriate inhibition of further pacing.

CASE 16 Onset of Ventricular Tachycardia during Pacemaker Threshold Testing

TEACHING POINTS
• PMT   • Troubleshooting
• Atrial undersensing

Case Presentation

The following tracing was obtained during threshold testing (Figure 1). You are urgently called for onset of VT during threshold testing. The setting is DDD at 90 beats/min.

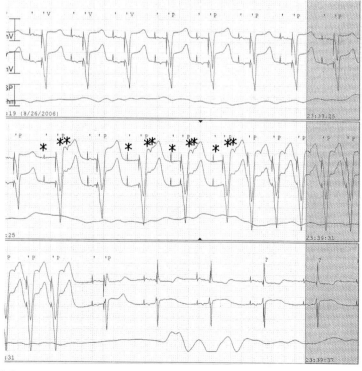

FIGURE 1

Case Discussion

What phenomenon is observed?

The top panel shows AV sequential pacing with capture of both chambers. In the middle panel, only the second atrial pacing spike captures the atrium (note absence of P waves, best seen on the bottom row of the middle panel, and corresponding retrograde P waves, manifested as a notch in the T wave of the top row of the middle panel).

After the first atrial spike in the middle panel, there is absence of further atrial spikes (arrow). Retrograde P waves (star), which could be seen earlier with each noncaptured atrial spike (double stars), are now sensed and tracked.

In the bottom panel, the third retrograde P wave is no longer tracked and the tachycardia terminates.

The absence of atrial capture is one of the causes of pacemaker-mediated tachycardia as subsequent ventricular paced impulses can conduct retrogradely via the AV node (because no atrial capture occurred, there was no penetration of the AV node and it can accommodate retrograde conduction).

Once enough delay in retrograde conduction occurs (after the sixth ventricular paced beat in the middle panel), the P waves fall outside of the postventricular atrial refractory period: it is sensed, tracked to the ventricle (because the AV node was just activated retrogradely, it is unlikely to accommodate antegrade conduction), by which time the node has recovered and able to assume retrograde conduction. A pacemaker mediated tachycardia (PMT) circuit is thus initiated and sustained.

Termination of PMT is due to an algorithm that prevents tracking of the atrial impulse after a predetermined number of Asense-Vpace events. This interrupts the "circuit" of PMT, terminating the tachycardia.

The abrupt onset of PMT should alert the physician to the possibility of atrial lead malfunction.

It should be kept in mind that both atrial noncapture (as described above) and atrial undersensing can lead to PMT. In the case of atrial undersensing, a P-wave is not tracked (because it is not sensed). Because a P wave is not sensed, the device follows with an atrial spike that usually does not capture (because the atrium is refractory because it was just activated by the intrinsic and undersensed P wave). Atrial noncapture follows, and the remainder of the mechanism of PMT initiation is as described above.

Management in this case is to make the atrial lead more sensitive by reprogramming or repositioning.

CASE 17 Dual-chamber Pacemaker with Possible Lead Malfunction

Case Presentation

The following tracings were recorded during routine telemetry (Figure 1). The patient had received a dual-chamber Medtronic pacemaker for sinus node dysfunction and intermittent AV block.

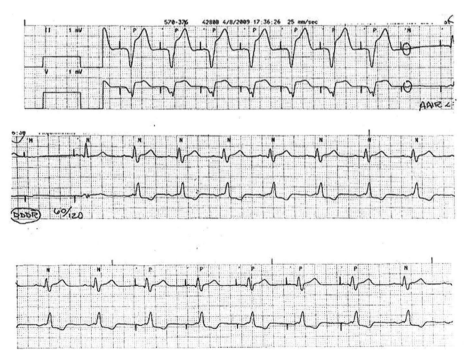

FIGURE 1

Case Discussion

What phenomenon is observed?

The top panel demonstrates AV sequential pacing for the first seven sequences. There is appropriate capture of the atrium and ventricle without evidence of atrial or ventricular noncapture. The eighth atrial paced impulse is not followed by ventricular pacing. The ninth paced atrial impulse (last impulse) is followed by intrinsic conduction.

The bottom panel, in essence, starts with the penultimate atrial paced impulse on the top panel. The first atrial impulse is nonconducted and not tracked. This may lead to the conclusion of ventricular oversensing by the ventricular lead. This is because the ventricular lead has inhibited pacing even though there is no ventricular activity.

The second atrial impulse is conducted via the native conduction system. Then, intrinsic sinus activity and native conduction take over. The first intrinsic QRS in the second panel is narrower than the subsequent ones (which appear to have incomplete right bundle branch morphology). In this case, intrinsic conduction occurs with appropriate inhibition of ventricular pacing. This rules out ventricular undersensing. The narrow initial QRS followed by slightly wider conducted impulses likely represents increased time for bundle branch recovery in the first conducted beat.

Although it may appear that there is device malfunction (specifically ventricular oversensing with inhibition of ventricular pacing), this algorithm is part of the managed ventricular pacing algorithm used in dual-chamber devices (implantable cardioverter defibrillators and pacemakers). Its underlying purpose is to minimize the amount of right ventricular pacing as it is thought that right ventricular pacing can be deleterious to myocardial function. The algorithm, in essence, gives the AV node every chance to conduct by transiently acting in a nontracking mode. In this situation, a paced or sensed atrial impulse does not initiate an AV timing interval. This allows maximum opportunity for the impulse to conduct to the ventricle. A blocked atrial beat is tolerated so long as the subsequent beat conducts.

These tracings demonstrate the latter finding, wherein the device allows native ventricular conduction even if it requires allowing a blocked atrial impulse for a single beat. In this case, this allowed recovery of conduction.

CASE 18   Inflammatory Reaction on Device Site

TEACHING POINTS

- Hypersensitivity to device composites
- Management of device allergy

Case Presentation

A 75-year-old white male was evaluated for swelling and redness over his pacemaker (PM) site. He was diagnosed with third-degree AV block and a permanent PM was implanted on his upper left chest two months earlier. He noted redness, pain, and swelling in the area of the PM three days before presentation. He denied any fever or chills but admitted to general weakness. Medical history was remarkable for diabetes, coronary heart disease, hyperlipidemia, and hypertension. He denied any allergy. He was a smoker and consumed alcohol socially. Medications include atorvastatin, lopressor, aspirin, and pioglitazone. Examination was remarkable for a low-grade fever, erythema, swelling, and mild tenderness over the PM site (Figure 1).

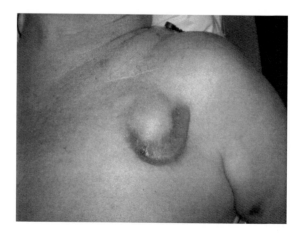

FIGURE 1

Case Discussion

The differential diagnoses for his presentation are mainly device infection and rarely allergic reaction to metal.

What to do next?

The patient was hospitalized with possible diagnosis of PM pocket infection. The PM generator was removed, a temporary PM was placed, and he was started on antibiotics.

The blood work, including complete blood count and electrolytes, were unremarkable. Transeshophageal echocardiogram was unremarkable for any vegetation. Two sets of blood cultures and the pocket swab culture remained negative after four days. The erythema and swelling improved.

What to do next?

- Implant a new generator on the right side and discharge him on antibiotics.

or

- Perform a skin patch test for metal allergy.

Infection is the most common cause of inflammation at implantable cardiac device sites. Although infection should be thoroughly investigated, an allergic reaction should be kept in mind (see Case 7, page 27). Previous studies have reported negative cultures in groups of patients with signs and symptoms of device infection, which are thought to be due to previous antibiotic use.

Hypersensitivity and allergic reactions to the metallic composite of implantable heart rhythm devices (IHRDs), including implantable cardiac defibrillators and pacemakers, are rare complications of IHRD implantation. Patients can present with local or systemic signs and symptoms of inflammation and /or device malfunction.

Different brands of IHRDs contain different composites, and these can be obtained from their vendors. Mainly, IHRD generators are covered with a titanium capsule. The header, where leads are attached to the generator, has two components: polymethylmethacrylate (the glassy part) and silicone rubber. The leads are composed of conductor wires and pacing or shock electrodes. The conducting wires are mainly composed of an alloy of Ni, Co, Cr, and Mo (MP35N) or MP35N with a silver core for high-current use. Pacing electrodes are made of platinum, platinuiridium, or tantalum with platinum coating. Some defibrillators may have a titanium shock coil, although these are not common.

Allergic reactions to IHRDs commonly present with dermatitis and pain over the implantation site from two days to two years after implantation. Rarely, it can also present as generalized puritis. Any of the metallic components can be the culprit. For instance, titanium allergy can be diagnosed by patch testing, lymphocyte proliferation tests, or intradermal test with serum contained titanium. The same methods can be used to test allergy to other components.

Management includes local steroid for mild dermatitis or removal of the device and implantation a new one without the causal composite. The successful use of gold- or silicone-coated devices and leads in prevention of sensitivity reaction has been reported previously. Custom-made IHRDs without allergen composite can be used for these patients.

IMPLANTABLE CARDIAC DEFIBRILLATORS

Implantable Cardiac Defibrillator Teaching Points (ICD)

CASE 1   Exercise-induced Implantable Cardioverter Defibrillator Shocks

TEACHING POINTS	
• Oversensing	• Double counting
• T-wave oversensing	• Blanking periods

Case Presentation

A 54-year-old man with a history of prior myocardial infarction presents with multiple ICD shocks, each occurring shortly after jogging.

The tracing below was obtained during interrogation of his device (Figure 1).

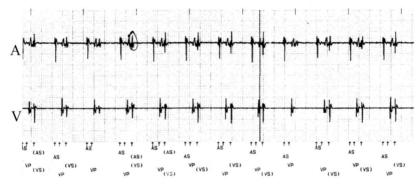

FIGURE 1

Case Discussion

What observations can be made?

The top channel (atrial) is followed by a far-field event that is not sensed.

The ventricular channel, however, demonstrates a ventricular paced event (no atrial signal is discernable) followed by a ventricular sensed event. The causes for a sensed event after a paced event include the following:

- Failure to capture and intrinsic conduction comes through.
- Premature ventricular contractions (PVCs).
- Intermyocardial or intrafascicular reentrant echo beats
- Capture latency giving rise to local myocardial capture beyond the ventricular blanking period
- Far-field signal from trans-septal myocardial activation

It should be noted that it is normal and expected for sensing to occur immediately after a paced beat, as tissue depolarization can last well beyond the duration of the stimulus artifact. To avoid this, devices have a blanking period programmed. This period is usually not programmable and can last anywhere between 20 and 200 msec for Medtronic devices, 125 to 157 msec for St. Jude devices (programmable), and 20 to 200 msec for Boston Scientific devices (programmable).

Is this a second ventricular event, independent from the ventricular pacing?

Two features make this unlikely: first, there is a fixed interval between the paced and the sensed event. Such fixed coupling may imply that the second (sensed) event is dependent on the paced event. Although a reentrant beat, for example, may be associated with a paced beat, this is somewhat unlikely in the current situation given the next observation. The very close coupling interval between the paced and the sensed events makes it physiologically less likely for the sensed event to be an independent impulse and strongly implies "double counting" of the paced beat. What has occurred is that the paced impulse has encountered delay in conduction to such an extent that ventricular myocardium is still being activated after the ventricular paced refractory period is over. The ventricular channel detects and senses this delayed activation as a ventricular sensed event.

Could this be T-wave oversensing?

This is not likely because the interval between the ventricular paced and sensed events is too short for the T wave to have occurred. Shortly after the first tracing, the following tracing is obtained (Figure 2).

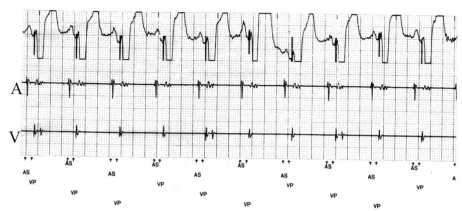

FIGURE 2

What observations can be made?

We now see that at a slower atrial sensed rate, ventricular paced events are not associated with a ventricular sensed event after ventricular pacing. A likely explanation is that as the rate slows down, the delay in ventricular conduction of the ventricular paced impulse lessens. At the faster rate, either the blanking period is shorter or the ventricular electrograms are occurring later. As discussed above, the absence of such a delay eliminates the substrate for double counting. Furthermore, at the faster rate, the first, third, and fifth beats on the atrial channel sense the ventricular paced beat. This may be because the delay in ventricular activation exceeds the post-ventricular atrial blanking period, a timing used in the atrial channel so that the paced ventricular beat is not sensed in the atrium (similar to the ventricular blanking period).

How would we manage this situation?

The most likely cause of this observation must be analyzed: based on the surface tracing, we know that ventricular capture occurs and that reentrant beats or PVCs do not follow. Sensing occurs before the T wave, ruling out T-wave oversensing. The regularity of the sensed event rules out noise. Thus, the most likely cause is local ventricular latency leading to sensing beyond the blanking period. A management strategy would be to increase the postpacing refractory period so that delayed activation due to pacing would be less likely to be sensed.

In the case of T-wave oversensing, double counting, or noise, another option would be to decrease the sensitivity of the ventricular lead. In this situation, one can *increase* the value, telling the pacemaker to ignore any signals smaller than the cutoff. By turning up the sensitivity parameter value, the device has become less sensitive because it is being instructed to ignore more signals. If you see only people taller than 6 ft 2 in (higher sensitivity setting), you will see less people than if you see people taller than 5 ft (lower sensitivity setting). Decreasing the device's sensitivity, however, may increase the probability of undersensing ventricular arrhythmias and should be done cautiously.

Multiple Implantable Cardioverter Defibrillator Shocks in a 45-year-old Man

TEACHING POINTS

- Inappropriate ICD shocks
- Arrhythmia detection algorithms

Case Presentation

A 45-year-old man presents with 13 ICD shocks, all of which occurred within a 5-min period.

The following tracings are obtained (Figure 1):

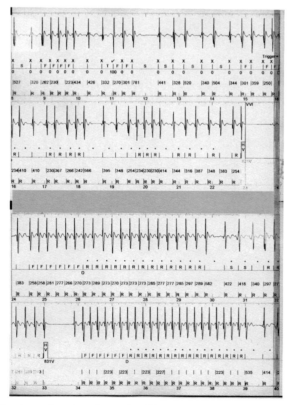

FIGURE 1 Tracings showing irregular V.

Case Discussion

What observations can be made?

The tracings demonstrate irregular ventricular activity. The morphology of the tracings remains unchanged during slower versus more rapid ventricular activity. These findings are highly suggestive of atrial fibrillation (AF) with rapid ventricular conduction as the etiology for the rapid ventricular activity. Because the conduction exceeds the cutoff for ventricular fibrillation detection, the device will ignore any other features (so-called discriminators, discussed below) used in determining whether to "declare" an episode. In this case, the device declares (erroneously) ventricular fibrillation and delivers a shock. What is more telling, however, is the rate of activation after the shock. Very rapid conduction of AF can be observed. In general, the more rapidly AF conducts, the less variability one observes between the beats. As such, one of the important discriminating features is rendered less useful. Furthermore, the 9th and 18th beats (star) are aberrantly conducted, rendering another discriminator (morphology).

Three common discriminators are commonly used to differentiate rapid ventricular conduction of supraventricular arrhythmias from true ventricular arrhythmia:

- **Morphology**: an algorithm performs a morphological analysis of the intracardiac electrograms. Similarity to baseline values argues against ventricular tachycardia (VT).
- **Stability**: variability in beat-to-beat intervals suggests atrial fibrillation with irregular ventricular conduction.
- **Onset**: sinus tachycardia usually presents with a gradual increase in heart rate. Thus, an onset that is not abrupt (gradual increase in rate) suggests sinus tachycardia.

There are two very important observations from this case: first, a shock is a very traumatic experience. There is a tremendous adrenergic response that leads, very often, to more rapid conduction of AF. This then leads to further shocks, followed by even more heightened anxiety, thus initiating a positive feedback loop that can lead to multiple ICD shocks. Second, when a patient complains of multiple shocks over a very brief period of time, there should be a high index of suspicion for inappropriate shocks.

CASE 3 Interrogation of a Dual-chamber Implantable Cardioverter Defibrillator

TEACHING POINTS

- Fusion
- Pseudofusion
- Noncapture

Case Presentation

The following tracing is obtained during routine interrogation of a dual-chamber ICD (Figure 1).

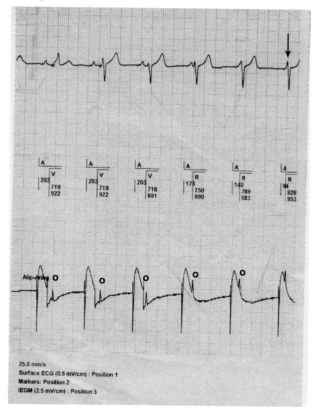

FIGURE 1

Case Discussion

What observations can be made?

The top line shows the surface ECG, the middle channel is the markers, and the bottom channel shows the atrial electrogram. "A" reflects atrial pacing, "R" is intrinsic ventricular activity, and "V" is a paced ventricular event.

The first beat shows an atrial paced event followed by what the device deems to be a ventricular paced event. Indeed, the ventricular pacing artifact can be observed on the atrial channel (asterisk). The surface QRS is different than the fourth, fifth, and sixth QRS morphologies, none of which are paced. Thus, this beat is, at least in part, paced. In the St. Jude devices, a paced impulse is noted by a V on the channel marker (A for the atrium), whereas an intrinsic ventricular beat is annotated by R (P for the atrium). Very importantly, the QRS morphology of the second beat is distinct from the first (paced) and identical to the last three impulses. We know that the last three impulses are not paced (the marker channels show R). Thus, the second beat, although marked as paced (V), is not paced. This phenomenon, wherein a paced stimulus never captures the chamber because it is preempted by intrinsic activation, is labeled **pseudofusion** (see below).

The third beat, however, shows an atrial paced event followed by a ventricular sensed event. The device has not delivered a pacing artifact, nor can one be seen on the atrial channel (as a far-field observation from the ventricular chamber). The QRS morphology, however, looks unchanged. The same phenomenon repeats itself in the fourth beat.

It can be concluded now that the ventricular chamber was never paced, as the QRS morphology between the paced and the nonpaced beats looks identical.

Do these observations signify ventricular noncapture?

Not necessarily. What is more likely occurring (although ventricular noncapture is still a possibility) is pseudofusion. In pseudofusion, a paced impulse is delivered, but this paced impulse does not contribute to myocardial activation. More often than not, the reason is simultaneous native conduction, which precludes the activation of that chamber by the pacing stimulus.

In the current tracing, it is likely that the ventricular activation of the first two beats were delayed just long enough for ventricular pacing to be delivered (by virtue of reaching the lower rate limit interval of the pacemaker). Antrioventricular (AV) conduction, however, preempted the ventricular paced artifact, and conduction occurred such that ventricular activation was not contributed to by the paced impulse.

The distinction between paced, fused (true combination of pacing and intrinsic activation), and pseudofusion has two clinical implications: in cardiac resynchronization therapy, the device interprets a pseudofused beat as a paced beat. This may erroneously overestimate the frequency of resynchronization. Pseudofusion is, in essence, pacing output without effective capture. This can lead to a drain on the battery.

Furthermore, both tracings demonstrate progressive shortening of AV intervals. The last three tracings show R waves that occur immediately after or simultaneously with the paced atrial impulse. This suggests that the R waves are not conducted. A rapid junctional rhythm may be operative.

As a final point, we have extended the tracing to show the impulse before the tracing above (arrow). Here, we can see atrial and ventricular pacing with a paced QRS morphology. This reinforces that pseudofusion, not ventricular noncapture, was operative above.

CASE 4   Long-QT Syndrome and Multiple Implantable Cardioverter Defibrillator Shocks

TEACHING POINTS

- Inappropriate ICD shocks
- Lead fracture
- Noise

Case Presentation

A 26-year-old with a single-chamber ICD because of inherited long-QT syndrome has 22 ICD shocks while dancing at a nightclub.

At the ER the following tracings are obtained (Figure 1):

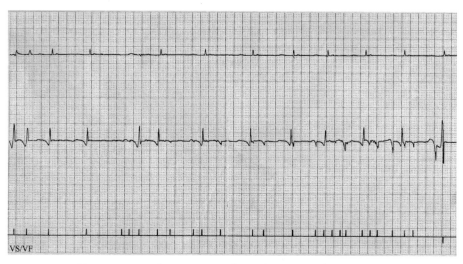

VS/VF

FIGURE 1 From top to bottom: surface electrocardiogram (ECG), electrogram, and electrogram marker channel. The electrograms are the far-field right ventricular lead (tip to coil).

Case Discussion

What caused the shocks?

The surface ECG demonstrates sinus rhythm with intrinsic conduction. The first two and the fifth beats are aberrantly conducted premature atrial contractions. This is reflected in the variation in the morphology of the corresponding intracardiac electrograms. The electrograms, however, demonstrate multiple signals not associated with any activity on the surface ECG. Importantly, the intervals of some of these signals (100 msec between the seventh and eighth signals on the marker channel) are at nonphysiological intervals. It is close to impossible to have ventricular recovery at such brief intervals. Some of the signals, therefore, do not reflect myocardial activity. If one traces each QRS from the surface ECG, regular activity associated with each QRS can be traced for both electrogram channels. These obviously represent true ventricular activation. The remaining do not.

What are the other sources of sensed activity as defined by the electrograms?

T-wave oversensing is possible but is not the case here, as many of the deflections do not coincide with the surface T waves. One would expect a regular interval between the actual sensed QRS and the oversensed T wave. This is not the case in the current tracing. Another possibility is oversensing due to potentially latent intrinsic depolarization ("QRS oversensing"). One of the causes may be a short postventricular blanking period. In this case, one would expect all "extra" electrograms to be associated with the surface QRS. This is not the case.

This leaves two other diagnostic possibilities: sensing of external noise (amplifiers in a nightclub) usually presents with signals of a regular frequency. This is not seen in this case. Still, the absence of these features does not rule out external noise because the source of the noise may have been irregular. The most likely explanation is lead or insulation fracture. Although each has unique findings, they can both present with what appears to be randomly sensed noise. Exceptions to this occur when the signals are filtered, as is the case with "noise reversion," wherein the device detects what it believes to be noise and filters it out. Blanking periods may also lend a regular pattern to irregular noise.

In the case of lead fracture, impedance to current flow is increased (since the current flow through the lead conductor), and pacing thresholds may be increased; with insulation failure, impedance is decreased (because the insulation to radial current flow is interrupted). Keep in mind that neither these findings may occur during device interrogation. Frequently, patients have to undergo provocative maneuvering of their arm and shoulder or the pocket itself prior to reproducing either the noise or the abnormal electrical parameters. Thus, it is the stored electrograms from the event as logged by the device that provide the most significant clues to the etiology of the fracture.

In this case, a lead fracture had occurred, probably during dancing. Because of the patient's age, the fractured lead was explanted and a new lead was placed.

CASE 5   Frequent Palpitations in a Patient with Implantable Cardioverter Defibrillator

TEACHING POINTS

- Arrhythmias diagnosis algorithm
- "Wobble" phenomenon

Case Presentation

A 64-year-old man with a dual-chamber ICD complains of frequent palpitations. Interrogation of the ICD demonstrates multiple episodes of tachycardia defined as ventricular tachycardia (VT) (fibrillation).

A representative tracing is shown below (Figure 1).

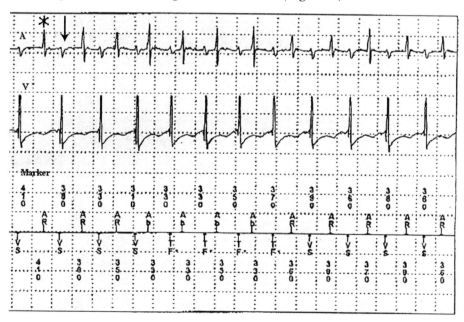

FIGURE 1   Top panel: atrial electrogram (A). Middle panel: ventricular electrogram (V). Bottom panel: marker channel (Marker).

Case Discussion

What is the likely rhythm?

The tachycardia demonstrates a regular pattern with 1:1 AV relationship. The differential includes SVT with rapid ventricular conduction versus VT with 1:1 VA conduction. The atrial electrogram shows a near-field atrial signal (star) followed by a far-field ventricular signal (arrow). This confirms the lead's position in the right arial appendage. The appendage drapes over the tricuspid valve. This accounts for the far-field ventricular signals.

With regard to the nature of the tachycardia, the most important observation is that of tachycardia "wobble." The concept of wobble is straightforward: During tachycardia, any alterations in cycle length will be initiated by the tachycardia "driver." Thus, alterations in A-A and V-V intervals will be first noted in the A-A interval if the tachycardia's genesis is the atrium (or, at least, not the ventricle). If the wobble is first noted in the V-V intervals, then the origin of the tachycardia is likely the ventricle and diagnosis will be VT (Figure 2).

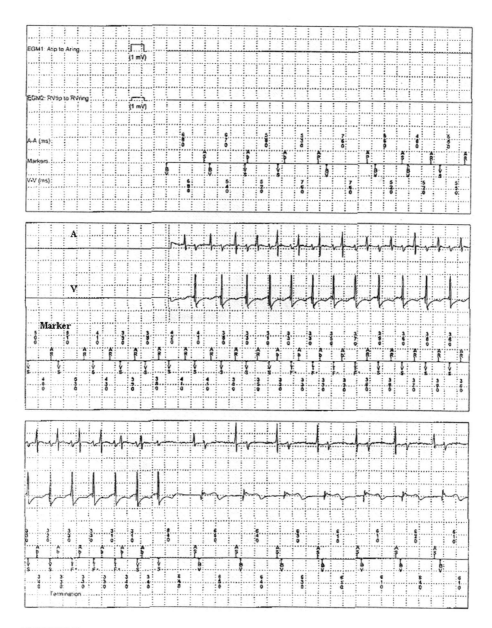

FIGURE 2

Turning our attention to the tracing, we can appreciate that A-A intervals of 410 and 390 msec are followed by V-V intervals of the same duration. This suggests supraventricular origin for the tachycardia. The next A-A interval, however, is 330 msec with a subsequent V-V interval of 350 msec. Why, if the tachycardia is originating above the ventricle, is the A-A interval of 330 msec not followed by an identical V-V interval? The answer lies in the fact that the AV node has decremental properties. Thus, the V-V interval during SVT may not be able to keep up with the increased atrial rate because of the delay in the AV node. The reverse of this is seen later when a 20 msec increase in the A-A (330 to 350 msec) leads to no change in the V-V interval (330 msec on consecutive V-Vs). The most likely explanation is that the delay in the A-A allows the AV node to recover enough to allow enhanced AV nodal conduction, which compensates for the delay. In other words, the 20 msec delay in the A-A interval has allowed the AV node to conduct 20 msec faster. The next effect is that the V-V interval remains unchanged at 330 msec.

This brings us to another important point: wobble is not necessarily reflected by *identical* changes in intervals. It is the trend in the alterations that is most important.

The next image (Figure 2) confirms two observations: (1) the tachycardia is *not* driven by the ventricle as the atrium is the chamber in which the tachycardia terminates first. This further reinforces the previous conclusion of SVT/AT as the tachycardia mechanism. (2) We can also see that the far-field deflection in the atrial channel is indeed due to ventricular activity.

Palpitations in a Patient with a Dual-chamber Implantable Cardioverter Defibrillator

---

TEACHING POINTS

- Atrial high-rate events
- Mode switching
- Pacing timing intervals

Case Presentation

A 64-year-old has a dual-chamber ICD (St Jude Current DR VT detection interval 300-400 msec; ventricular fibrillation (VF) detection interval at a cycle length (CL) <300 msec). On routine office visit, she was noted to complain of intermittently irregular pulse. Interrogation of her ICD demonstrated the following tracing (Figure 1):

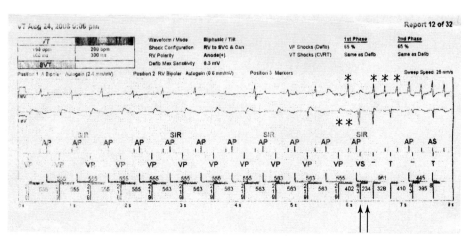

FIGURE 1 Top to bottom: atrial electrograms, ventricular electrograms, channel marker (A and V).

Case Discussion

What is the diagnosis? What can be a contributing factor to this diagnosis? How would you reprogram the device to prevent this from occurring?

The device demonstrates ventricular paced events followed by atrial events (asterisk), which are noted on the channel marker (arrow) but are not detected. This is followed by an atrial pacer artifact seen both on the channel marker (double asterisk) and the atrial electrogram (double arrow). It does not capture the atrium, likely because the atrium is refractory. This is followed by irregular, rapid atrial activation representing atrial flutter or fibrillation. The ventricular response also becomes irregular and rapid, in line with rapid ventricular conduction of Atrial fibrillation (AF). The rate toward the end of the tracing becomes so rapid that some beats are diagnosed as ventricular tachycardia. In this case, the first part of the tracing demonstrates ventricular pacing, which is likely due to the tracking of a noncaptured Apace (note that Apace-Vpace rates and intervals are regular and identical [555 and 219 msec, respectively] at the beginning of the tracing). This rules out pacemaker-mediated tachycardia (ie, Vpace in response to Asense).

Why is the patient having atrial pacing in the setting of Asense events?

This is a feature of the device used to prevent AF by overdrive pacing the atrium during atrial high rates. Some studies have suggested that acceleration in atrial pacing rates after atrial ectopy may be protective with regard to AF induction. The rationale is that immediate acceleration in pacing leads to overdrive suppression of imminent AF, in essence terminating the AF before its onset. It is, however, possible that such acceleration in pacing can itself be proarrhythmic.

In this case, the Apace does not capture, but the Vpace does. As the Apace is occurring, atrial ectopy, the first beats of which are not sensed (triple asterisk), can be noted with conversion to a more rapid atrial event. The initial atrial events, which are noted by the marker channel but not annotated, are within the refractory period of the atrial channel (postventricular atrial refractory period). Thus, an immediate Apace (and ensuing

Vpace) is delivered. If the postventricular atrial refractory period were to be shortened, then the true atrial events would be sensed and the immediately following Apace event would not occur. Whether this would prevent atrial acceleration is less certain because there does not appear to be an Apace that captures and triggers atrial acceleration.

CASE 7   Variable Pacing in a Patient with Congenital Atrioventricular Block

TEACHING POINTS

- Variable atrial pacing
- Total atrial refractory period (TARP)

Case Presentation

The following electrocardiogram is obtained in a patient with a dual-chamber ICD (DDDR, 60–140 beats/min). She has congenital complete heart block.

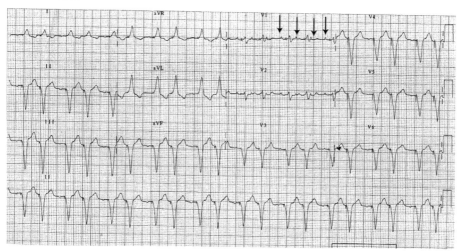

FIGURE 1

Case Discussion

What observations can be made?

The ventricular rhythm is paced. Regular, periodic alteration in the ventricular rate is noted: every other paced impulse has an equal and shorter coupling interval. The alternating intervals are equal (400 and 600 msec).

The atrial rhythm is regular with P waves best seen on lead V_1 (arrows) and can also be seen in lead II (arrows). The P waves occur at a CL of 360 msec. Their morphology is suggestive of a left atrial tachycardia (upright in V_1).

Closer inspection of lead V_1 demonstrates the periodic nature of the AV relationship. Starting with the first arrow, the P wave is sensed and an AV interval of 180 msec leads to ventricular tracking. The subsequent P waves are sensed. However, the AV interval has to be prolonged to accommodate the upper rate limit of 140 beats/min. The third P wave occurs during the postventricular refractory blanking period and is not tracked. The cycle repeats itself.

The atrial tachycardia does not lead to mode switching because the atrial rate is 167 beats/min, and the high-rate definition is set at 170 beats/min.

Upper rate behavior refers to the pattern of AV conduction during an atrial sensed rate that exceeds the upper tracking rate of the pacemaker. An assumption is that intrinsic AV conduction does not occur. There are essentially three patterns: one is group beating as demonstrated above. The second is prompt reversion to 2:1 AV block. This occurs when the total atrial refractory period, which is defined as the postatrial refractory period plus the programmed sensed AV interval, is greater than the sensed atrial cycle length. Finally, Wenckebach periodicity may occur if the total atrial refractory period is less than the sensed atrial cycle length. The Wenckebach is not typical in that the ventricular interval is regular (at the upper rate limit of the pacemaker).

CASE 8 Multiple Implantable Cardioverter Defibrillator Shocks

TEACHING POINTS

- T-wave oversensing
- Sensing
- Double counting
- Arrhythmia-detection algorithms
- Device troubleshooting

Case Presentation

A patient with a dual-chamber ICD presents with multiple shocks. Interrogation of the episodes is shown below (Figure 1).

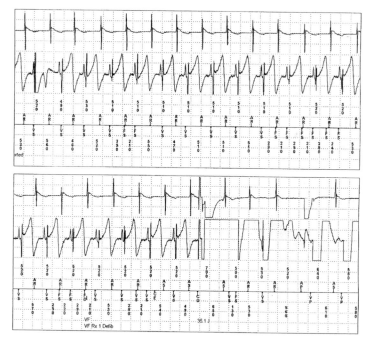

FIGURE 1 Top panel: atrial electrogram. Middle panel: right ventricular (RV) tip/RV ring electrogram. Bottom panel: marker channel.

Case Discussion

What is the cause of implantable cardioverter defibrillator shocks?

What treatment options may be offered?

The first three impulses demonstrate AV sensing without any abnormalities. After the fourth sensed atrial event, however, the T wave of the corresponding QRS was sensed. Note that the RV signals grossly demonstrate large T waves. This T-wave oversensing then caused inappropriate detection of VF and inappropriate ICD shock. Note that after the ICD shock is delivered, most ICDs are programmed to perform high output pacing. This then eliminates the T-wave oversensing as no intrinsic QRS conduction occurs.

The patients presenting electrogram in the clinic is show below:

It can be appreciated that T-wave oversensing is not a continuous problem.

In fact, the patient demonstrated T-wave oversensing *only* when his sinus rate approached 110 beats/min (note that the sinus CL was 510 msec [117 beats/min] during the T-wave oversensing episode).

We elected to increase the patient's β-blockade because this finding was associated with rate-dependent aberrancy in ventricular conduction. Another option would have been making the RV lead less sensitive. Given the size of the T waves during the episode (they approached the R waves), it was thought this may not be effective and it may compromise detection of VT/VF (by leading to undersensing). The final, invasive option would have been to reposition the RV lead or implant an RV pace/sense lead (smaller caliber). The latter would preclude the need for removal of the chronically implanted lead because sensing would occur via the new lead and therapies would be delivered via the chronic lead.

T-wave oversensing should not be confused with "double counting" of the QRS by the device. In the case of the latter, the ICD senses two components for each QRS (not the T wave). The sensed components may vary, and thus, a regular coupling interval between sensed beats may not necessarily be seen.

CASE 9 Rapid Analysis of Shock Etiology

TEACHING POINTS

- T-wave oversensing
- Double counting
- Inappropriate ICD shocks
- Lead malfunction
- Device diagnostics

Case Presentation

A patient with a dual-chamber ICD presents with a shock.

You are privy to only the following graph (Figure 1):

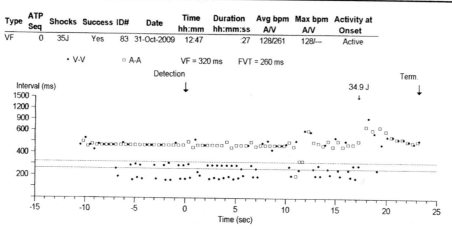

Type	ATP Seq	Shocks	Success	ID#	Date	Time hh:mm	Duration hh:mm:ss	Avg bpm A/V	Max bpm A/V	Activity at Onset
VF	0	35J	Yes	83	31-Oct-2009	12:47	:27	128/261	128/---	Active

FIGURE 1

Case Discussion

What is the diagnosis?

The diagram demonstrates ventricular (dark boxes) and atrial (light boxes) intervals.

The x-axis shows time progression during the episode and demonstrates the event before (negative time), during, and after the episode.

The y-axis demonstrates corresponding intervals in msec between atrial or ventricular events.

The horizontal lines demonstrate the cutoff (in msec) for detection of ventricular tachycardia and fibrillation (top and bottom lines, respectively).

On the right, corresponding A and V events at identical intervals can be seen. There is a sudden decrease in the V-V intervals such that they are clustered in alternate cycle lengths of around 300 and 200 msec.

This is characteristic for *both* T-wave oversensing and "double counting" of the QRS. The salient feature is that there are two alternating populations of intervals.

This is to be expected for both T-wave oversensing and double counting of QRS because each actual QRS is sensed as two events. Assuming that these events are the same (which it always is for T-wave oversensing as the device senses the QRS and T waves and usually, but not always, is the case for double counting), a regular interval will be observed between events. Because of this, a fixed coupling interval of alternating sensed events will be noted on the graph.

True ventricular tachycardia rarely presents with alternating cycle lengths (although this not theoretically impossible).

In fact, this graph was obtained from the patient in the previous case.

In this case, simple pattern recognition can assist in making the correct diagnosis.

CASE 10 Wide Complex Tachycardia with Periodic Oscillation

Case Presentation

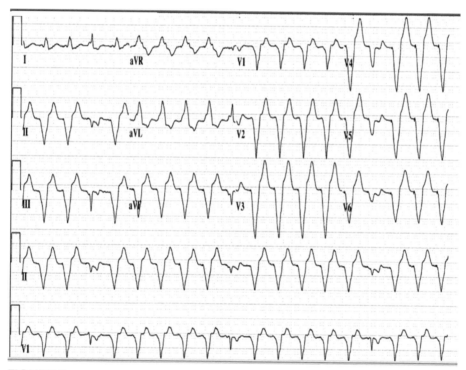

FIGURE 1

Case Discussion

The 12-lead demonstrates a regular wide complex tachycardia in a patient with a dual-chamber ICD (DDDR, 50-120 beats/min).

Why did the implantable cardioverter defibrillator not deliver therapy?

The electrocardiogram shows a regular wide complex tachycardia. The 3rd, 9th, and 15th ventricular complexes are narrow and are preceded by small P waves with a fixed AV coupling.

It is possible that the tracing shows ventricular tachycardia (VT) with fusion beats (between VT and sinus capture of the ventricle with intrinsic ventricular conduction. Assuming this to be the case we have a situation where the degrees of fusion are identical since the morphologies are identical). Because fusion beats during VT are a result of ventricular activation via both VT and intrinsic ventricular activation, their morphologies often vary, and because the relative contributions of each factor (VT and intrinsic conduction) can be variable, the morphologies of fusion beats are often dissimilar. In the current tracing, we see that all three beats have identical morphologies. The odds of fusion beats being so similar is not high and argues against these being fusion beats.

Another observation is that the P waves do not appear to be sinus in origin, as they are quite flat in the inferior leads and have no terminal negative forces in lead V_1.

A final observation is that the tachycardia is 120 beats/min, exactly same as the upper tracking rate of the ICD.

The patient was in atrial tachycardia with a rate of 120 beats/min. The atrial rhythm was not fast enough to cause mode switch to a nontracking pacing mode. The device was simply tracking this left sided atrial tachycardia.

During the three conducted beats, the AV node conducted rapidly enough to preempt ventricular pacing.

Interestingly, there seems to be a regular conducted interval of every sixth conducted beat. It is possible that this reflects the periodicity by which time the AV node has acquired adequate recovery to allow rapid AV conduction and, therefore, preemption of ventricular pacing.

CASE 11   Ventricular Ectopy on a Rhythm Strip

TEACHING POINTS

- Detection algorithms
- Morphology
- Sensing

Case Presentation

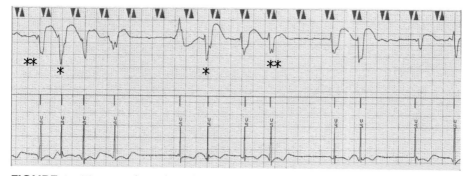

FIGURE 1 Top panel: surface rhythm strip. Middle panel: marker channel. Bottom panel: electrogram channel.

What observations can be made?

The surface tracings show runs of ventricular tachycardia (VT) at a relatively slow rate. The important observation is that the morphology of the VT is variable (polymorphic). Each morphology, however, has a corresponding intracardiac morphology.

The second and sixth QRS morphologies, for example, are similar. The corresponding intracardiac electrograms show an initial marked upstroke followed immediately by a second, smaller upstroke (star). This observation cannot be made for any of the other QRS morphologies.

The first and eighth QRS morphologies are also similar. The corresponding intracardiac electrograms show a terminal, sharp, negative force (double star).

These features may be incorporated into "morphology" algorithms that may allow discrimination of suplaveotricular tachycardia (SVT) from VT.

In these algorithms, the device will initially define what the "normal" morphology of the ventricular signal looks like. Typically, a relatively far-field vector (such as right ventricular coil to right ventricular tip) will be used (template). Specific levels of alteration to the template will then be noted by the device.

Deviations from cutoffs (usually programmable) will lead the device to define the morphology of the tachycardia to be variable enough so as to "declare" VT.

A potential pitfall of such algorithms may be that they fail to recognize rate-dependent aberrancy during SVT and rapid ventricular conduction. This feature can be active or "passive," in which case it will not contribute to detection of VT.

CASE 12   Ventricular Pacing and Atrial Flutter

TEACHING POINTS

- Mode switching
- Sensing
- Tracking
- Atrial tachyarrhythmias
- Upper rate behavior

Case Presentation

The following electrocardiogram is obtained from a dual-chamber ICD (Figure 1).

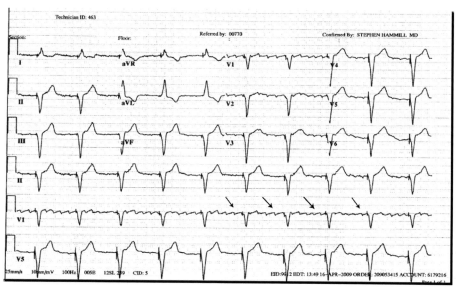

FIGURE 1

Case Discussion

What observations can be made?

A regularly paced ventricular rhythm is observed. There is no atrial pacing. There are no conducted atrial impulses. These findings suggest that there is appropriate ventricular pacing, although one cannot comment on ventricular sensing because of the absence of intrinsic ventricular activation.

With regard to the atrial lead, the atrial rhythm is rapid, regular, without any apparent isoelectric periods (best seen on lead V_1) and suggests atrial flutter. Thus, it appears that atrial sensing is preserved since there is inhibition of atrial pacing for the duration of the electrocardiogram.

The ventricular rhythm is paced and regular.

Close inspection demonstrates that there is no fixed relationship between the atrial flutter waves and the ventricular pacing spikes. This is a very important observation and suggests that atrial sensing does *not* lead to the initiation of an AV interval. If it had, a fixed interval between the flutter waves and the ventricular pacing spikes would be observed. This is not seen (look at the rhythm strip for lead V_1 and note that the interval between the ventricular spike and previous P wave occurs in different phases of the P wave) (arrows). The critical implication is that the pacemaker is not in a tracking mode.

The atrial lead has sensed the rapid atrial activation and initiated mode switch, during which the device reverts to a nontracking mode (VVI or VVIR).

The ventricle is then paced regularly without any consideration of atrial activity.

This observation of course requires absence of intrinsic flutter conduction. Were that to occur, ventricular pacing would be inhibited.

CASE 13 Ventricular Tachycardia Undersensing in a Dual-chamber Implantable Cardioverter Defibrillator

Case Presentation

The following strip was obtained during routine telemetry of a patient with a dual-chamber ICD (Figure 1). You were called for evaluation of device malfunction due to undersensing of ventricular tachycardia (VT).

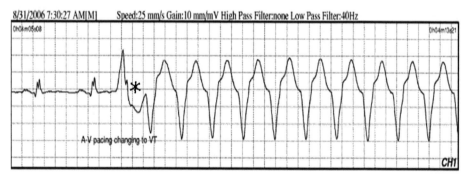

8/31/2006 7:30:27 AM[M]   Speed:25 mm/s Gain:10 mm/mV High Pass Filter:none Low Pass Filter:40Hz

0h04m05s08   0h04m13s21

A-V pacing changing to VT

CH1

FIGURE 1

Case Discussion

What observations can be made?

The first two beats demonstrate intrinsic P and QRS waves. No pacing is performed. This observation suggests that there is appropriate sensing of both the atrial and the ventricular leads because intrinsic activity was associated with the suppression (inhibition) of pacing. The third beat is a relatively late coupled PVC, which then leads to a regular, wide complex tachycardia. This may raise concern for undersensing of VT by this dual-chamber ICD. This is less likely, however, because at least during sinus rhythm, ventricular pacing was inhibited. As noted above, this indicates that the ventricular lead is at least sensing some ventricular activity. The other possibility is that the rate of the VT is below the cutoff for detection by the ICD.

Interrogation of the ICD demonstrated that what had happened in fact was that the PVC had led to a retrograde P wave (star) via the AV node. Because the beat immediately prior to the PVC had conducted down the AV node, the node was still relatively (but not absolutely) refractory. Thus, the retrograde P-wave conduction occurred with a marked delay. This delay caused the P wave to be so late so as to occur after the postventricular refractory period had timed out. Thus, the P wave was sensed.

The AV node, however, having just accepted retrograde conduction, was still in its absolute refractory period and the P wave could not travel back down the node. This caused the AV timing interval to time out. Ventricular pacing ensued. By this time, the node had recovered, and the paced ventricular impulse conducted back up the AV node. This demonstrates yet another mechanism by which pacemarker mediated tachycardia (PMT) can be initiated. A PVC is thus one of the most common causes of PMT initiation. This usually occurs in a PVC that has an intermediate coupling interval with the previous conducted QRS. Early PVCs are usually blocked in the retrograde direction in the AV node. Late PVCs conduct retrogradely rapidly enough so that the retrograde P wave occurs before the postventricular atrial refractory period times out. This, of course, will preempt tracking of the P wave to the atrium as the device will "ignore" the P wave.

CASE 14   A 52-year-old Man with a Beeping Implantable Cardioverter Defibrillator

<table>
<tr><td colspan="2" align="center">**TEACHING POINTS**</td></tr>
<tr><td>• Audible alerts</td><td>• Device troubleshooting</td></tr>
</table>

Case Presentation

A 52-year-old man complains of a "beeping" sound emanating from his ICD. He received the ICD two years earlier because of severe cardiomyopathy and ventricular tachycardia (VT). Nine months earlier, he had undergone placement of a left ventricular mechanical assistant pump. Three months earlier, he presented with multiple ICD shocks. Interrogation of the device had shown appropriate shocks which had successfully terminated frequent episodes of VT. The patient had been placed on three different antiarrhythmic medications, all of which failed to control his VT. The ICD shocks were severely debilitating. Because the patient's systemic circulation was a function of the left ventricular mechanical assistant pump and after discussion with the patient and his heart failure specialist, a decision was made to turn off ICD therapies.

Later on the day in which the therapies were turned off, the patient noticed an audible tone emanating from the ICD (Medtronic Inc., St. Paul, MN). The tone is described as alternating low and high pitch.

Medtronic

Parameters

Device: Concerto™ C154DWK

Data Collection Setup

Stored EGM

	EGM 1 (A or V)	EGM 2 (V)
EGM Source	Can to RVcoil	LVtip To RVcoil
EGM Range	+/- 8 mV	+/- 8 mV
Pre-arrhythmia EGM		Off

Additional Setup

Device Date/Time	21-Dec-2009 17:40
Holter Telemetry	Off
LECG Range	+/- 2 mV
V. Senses to Detect	10 senses
V. Paces to Terminate	3 paces

Medtronic CareAlert Setup

Patient Home Monitor	No
Alert Time	10:00

Alert Conditions	Enable-Urgency Tone	Threshold
AT/AF Daily Burden Settings	Off	6 hr
Avg. V. Rate During AT/AF Settings	Off	6 hr at 100 bpm
Number of Shocks Delivered in an Episode	Off	
All Therapies in a Zone Exhausted	Off	
A. Pacing Lead Impedance Out of Range	Off	
RV Pacing Lead Impedance Out of Range	On-High	<200 or >2500 ohms
LV Pacing Lead Impedance Out of Range	On-High	<200 or >2500 ohms
RV Defibrillation Lead Impedance Out of Range	On-High	<20 or >200 ohms
SVC Defib Lead Impedance Out of Range	On-High	<20 or >200 ohms
Low Battery Voltage RRT	On-High	2.62 V(RRT)
Excessive Charge Time EOS	On-High	
VF Detection OFF, 3+ VF or 3+ FVT Rx Off.	On-High	

Auto Cap Formation

Minimum Auto Cap Formation Interval	Auto

Last Charge to Full Energy

21-Dec-2009 09:06:36

Last Capacitor Formation

03-Dec-2008 20:44:31

FIGURE 1

Case Discussion

What are the causes of alternating implantable cardioverter defibrillator tones?

The most common cause of such tones is a low battery. The beeping usually occurs when the battery has arrived at its elective replacement indicator. This implies about three more months of longevity. Another cause of an alternating beeping sound may be abnormally high or low impedances. The latter can be seen with lead fractures or loose set screws in the header of the ICD, the former with insulation failure. Recent algorithms to detect fracture in the Sprint Fidelis Medtronic ICD lead incorporate high impedances with nonphysiological sensing (ie, coupling intervals between sensed events <150 msec) and have been integrated to cause the alternating "siren-like" tone. Noise reversion refers to the ICD's interpretation of noise and is another cause. Finally, when the ICD is programmed to turn off therapies, an alert will sound.

In the above cases, the alert usually occurs at a specific time of day and will repeat itself each day. The trigger for the alert is programmable. In the case of the above patient, the ICD was beeping because arrhythmia therapies had been turned off but the feature for audible alerts in such a circumstance had not been turned off. The patient had to visit the clinic where the feature was turned off.

A continuous audible alert can be heard when the ICD is exposed to a magnetic field. Of course, in this situation, the ICD will not be delivering therapies because of exposure to the field. This does not indicate device malfunction. A continuous audible tone is also a means for the patient or health care provider to be made aware of the possible effects of such exposure (inhibition of therapy).

In other cases, a continuous audible tone indicates that the device is functioning normally. In the case of the Medtronic Marquis premature battery depletion, this tone reassures the patient that there is no evidence of this process (programmable for these patients).

BIVENTRICULAR DEVICE TROUBLESHOOTING

BIVENTRICULAR TEACHING POINTS (BiV)

Case Series 1 Biventricular Device Troubleshooting

TEACHING POINTS

- Atrial lead
- Locating LV pacing lead
- Not allowing cardiac resynchronization
- Offset

Case 1.1 Locating the Left Ventricular Pacing Lead—Electrocardiographic Fluoroscopic Correlation

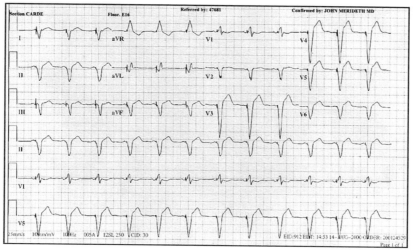

FIGURE 1

Biventricular (BiV) pacing systems have the right ventricular (RV) lead usually in the region of the RV apex. The left ventricular (LV) lead location is variable, with lead placement in the anterior, lateral, or posterior coronary venous systems. The electrocardiogram (EKG) in Figure 1 is obtained from a patient with a BiV system, and capture has been ascertained from both leads.

Where is the likely location of the left ventricular pacing lead?

    A) The LV lead is not capturing

    B) The anterior interventricular vein

    C) An anterolateral vein

    D) A posterolateral vein

    E) The middle cardiac vein

Answer D: A posterolateral vein

The R wave (right bundle branch block morphology) in lead V_1 suggests LV pacing. In addition, the QS complex in lead I is consistent with the stimulation site being in the left lateral wall (vector away from lead I, a left lateral lead). Having now deduced the pacing site to be in the LV and lateral wall, the finding of QS complexes in the inferior leads (II, III, and aVF) places the stimulation site and location of the LV pacing lead in the posterolateral location.

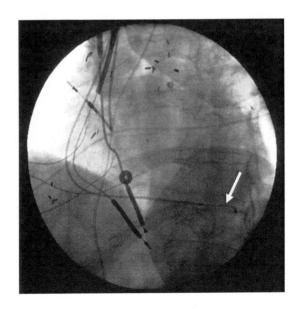

FIGURE 2

One must always correlate electrocardiography with fluoroscopy, and in most cases, exact knowledge and analysis of one will allow deduction of the other. For example, Figure 2 shows the left anterior oblique projection in a patient with an atrial lead, two implantable cardioverter defibrillator leads in the RV, and a single LV pacing lead (arrow). This lead is on the LV free wall and posterior. If such a fluoroscopic image was available and the pacing vector was anything different from that seen in Figure 1, then the physician should be alerted to either failure to capture or one of the other reasons described below for a potential malfunction of the system.

The following EKG was obtained from a patient who has a functional cardiac resynchronization therapy system. The LV thresholds are excellent. By reviewing the electrogram, what can be deduced in terms of likely causes for this patient not improving after implantation? The EKG was obtained during device interrogation with BiV stimulation and maximal output on the LV lead.

The reader should make a short list of possible causes for the patient's failure to improve before reading further.

Specific points that should be looked for during device interrogation or electrocardiography are the following:

- Is there LV capture?
- Where is the LV lead placed, and is that an appropriate location?
- Is there an appropriate offset between the LV and RV leads?
- Is the atrioventricular (AV) timing appropriate?
- Are there premature ventricular contraction (PVCs) that are present, and could they be affecting response, and others?

We have briefly examined the issue of appropriate placement of the LV lead in Figure 1. Let us now assess for appropriate RV-LV offset.

Case 1.2 Will Offset Help?

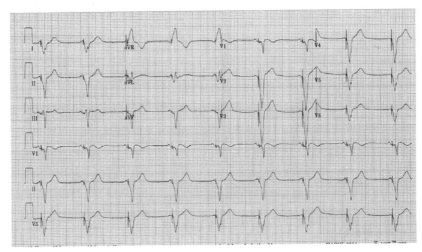

FIGURE 3 Biventricular pacing, 0 msec offset.

The electrocardiogram above is consistent with

A) Left ventricular pacing alone

B) Failure to capture on the ventricular lead

C) Right ventricular apical pacing alone

D) Predominant right ventricular pacing with minimal left ventricular lead contribution

E) Predominant left ventricular pacing with minimal right ventricular apical lead contribution

Answer D: Predominant right ventricular pacing with minimal left ventricular lead contribution

In Figure 3, an electrocardiogram from another patient with a BiV system and failure to improve is shown. Both LV and RV leads pace simultaneously; that is, there is no offset between the two. Left bundle branch morphology and QS complexes in leads II, III, and aVF are seen. This is very similar to what one expects from RV apical pacing. It is possible for the physician to assume that the LV lead is not capturing, although the QS complex in lead I suggests *some* LV stimulation contributing to cardiac activation.

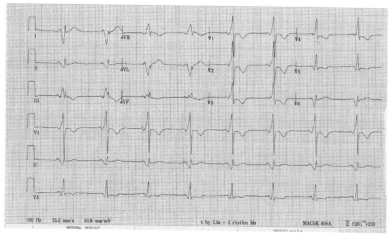

FIGURE 4

Figure 4, however, clearly shows that LV lead function is normal. Pacing from the LV lead alone is shown with the characteristic right bundle branch block morphology, and the slight positivity in leads III and aVF suggests a lateral (slightly anterior) location for the LV lead, generally an ideal and strived for placement site.

Why then does the vector seem entirely like right ventricular pacing when the right ventricular and left ventricular leads pace simultaneously (Figure 3)?

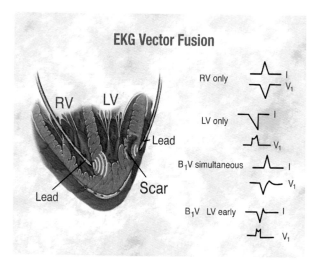

FIGURE 5 From Asirvatham (J Cardiovasc Electrophysiol. 2007;18:1028–1031).

Figure 5 illustrates the principle behind RV-LV offset programming based on the EKG. Even though both leads pace simultaneously, because there is a scar and relatively diseased tissue *near* the LV pacing site, the BiV simultaneous EKG looks very much like RV pacing alone. Because of the exit delay from the LV pacing lead, global ventricular activation is nearly completed by the RV pacing lead alone, and it is as if the LV lead is not there or not working. To compensate for this exit delay, the LV lead should be programmed to pace earlier than the RV lead (LV-RV offset). By programming an appropriately early offset (which will vary from patient to patient), near simultaneous and equal contribution of both leads to ventricular activation can occur.

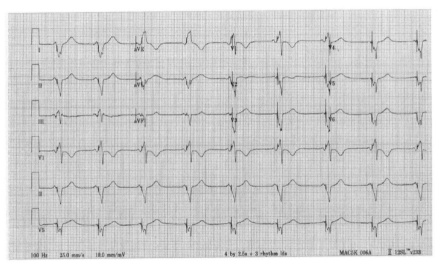

FIGURE 6   LV earlier than RV by 30 msec.

In Figure 6, the LV lead is programmed to pace about 30 msec before the RV lead. Now, we see a vector that is approximately a fusion between RV and LV pacing vectors. The R wave is more prominent in V_1 and the QS complex in lead III is no longer seen.

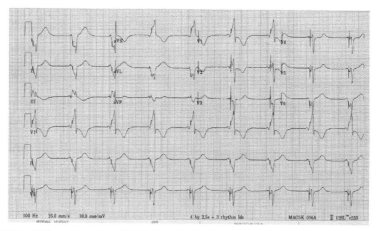

FIGURE 7 LV earlier than RV by 50 msec.

In Figure 7, the offset is now programmed even earlier (50 msec LV early). Now, the EKG looks very similar to LV pacing alone and there is little contribution from RV pacing, and it is now as if the RV pacing lead is not there or not working. The patient wound up having the offset programmed at 30 msec with significant improvement in heart failure symptoms.

Case 1.3 Not Allowing Cardiac Resynchronization

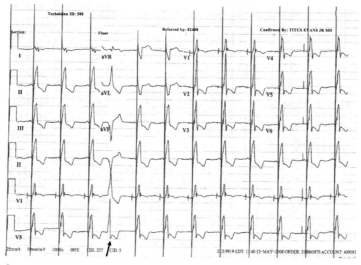

FIGURE 8

In the electrocardiogram obtained above, there appears to be excellent biventricular stimulation. The fourth beat appears to be excellent biventricular stimulation. What is represented by the fourth beat on this tracing (arrow)?

A) Loss of LV capture

B) Loss of RV capture

C) Intrinsic conduction

D) A right ventricular PVC

E) A left ventricular PVC

Answer E: A left ventricular PVC

Let us go back now to our initial patient (Figure 8). Here, the pacing vector seems reasonably consistent with BiV stimulation. A right bundle morphology is seen, however, with an isoelectric deflection in lead I (usually negative with LV pacing, usually positive with RV pacing alone). We should therefore look for other findings. We note that there is a PVC found on this random EKG. How could PVCs potentially affect clinical benefit from BiV stimulation?

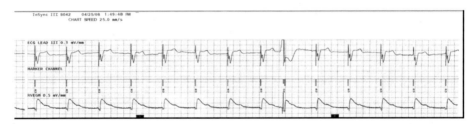

FIGURE 9

In Figure 9, one of the reasons why PVCs may cause failure to improve after BiV implantation is illustrated. When the PVC occurs, LV pacing may be inhibited, and thus, with frequent PVCs, the percentage of BiV pacing of all ventricular depolarizations may fall significantly below the desired 100% value. Biventricular output may still occur, but with failure to capture because most PVCs arise from the LV but sensing is from the RV (most devices). Thus, pseudofusion may occur. True fusion may also result if the PVC occurs simultaneous to BiV pacing stimulus. In either case (fusion or pseudofusion), ventricular stimulation is not truly BiV, yet on device interrogation, "100% BiV pacing" may be found.

Sometimes, a single PVC may result in continued inhibition of BiV pacing. The first PVC will inhibit BiV pacing, but the postventricular atrial refractory period (possibly lengthened by postventricular atrial refractory period extension if that feature is programmed on) will result in failure to sense a sinus beat if intrinsic sinus node function is present and the sinus rates are relatively fast. If intrinsic AV nodal conduction is also present, then the P wave that fell in the refractory period will result in a ventricular sensed event that again causes inhibition of BiV pacing, and the situation can perpetuate with lengthy periods of inhibited BiV pacing.

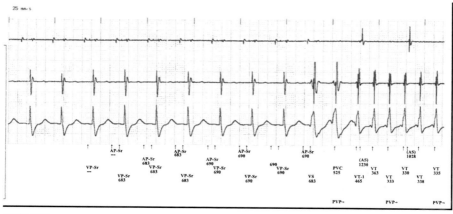

FIGURE 10

Analysis of PVCs and correlating with intracardiac device retrieved electrograms on interrogation can be helpful for further patient management. In the tracing seen in Figure 10, onset of ventricular tachycardia is noted. Each episode appeared to start with a very similar premature ventricular beat. Note that the near-field electrogram (middle line) starts later than the onset of the far-field electrogram (lower line). This suggests that early activation is in the LV (near-field electrogram from the RV pacing tip). The PVCs seen were also from the LV, suggesting that PVCs start tachycardia and could potentially be targeted for radiofrequency ablation. Note also that nonsustained VT will inhibit BiV pacing, and in this case, sinus rhythm (as a result of retrograde AV block) occurs (see atrial electrograms) and the patient can be symptomatic from the rapid beats, inhibition of BiV pacing, and atrioventricular dyssynchrony (pacemaker syndrome).

Case 1.4 Role of the Atrial Lead

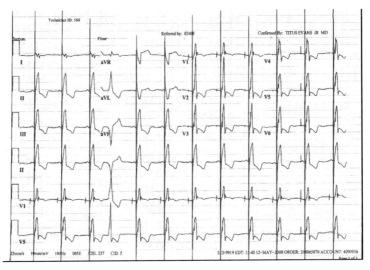

FIGURE 11

In the electrocardiogram shown in Figure 11, what can you say about the atrial lead?

A) There is no atrial capture

B) There is intrinsic sinus rhythm

C) The atrial lead is probably in the right atrial appendage

D) The atrial lead is probably in the vein of Marshall pacing the left atrium

E) The atrial lead is in the region of Bachmann's bundle

Answer C: The atrial lead is probably in the right atrial appendage

Let us get back to our original case discussion reproduced here in Figure 11. Is there atrioventricular synchrony? At first glance, we see AV sequential pacing with clear evidence of atrial capture (P wave after the atrial spikes in Figure 11). However, the caregiver needs to ascertain whether the atrial lead is appropriately placed and whether mechanical atrioventricular synchrony is likely to occur. The AV timing appears to be short, with the ventricular pacemaker spike occurring even before completion of the P wave. In traditional dual-chamber pacing systems (right atrium [RA]–RV), the AV interval is a good surrogate for left atrial (LA)–LV mechanical contraction intervals (synchrony). The atrial lead stimulates the RA first, and the activation wavefront then proceeds to the LA via Bachmann bundle. In the meanwhile, after the programmed AV delay, RV stimulation occurs and activation proceeds to the LA; thus, LA-LV intervals are similar to what one would predict from the programmed AV interval. With BiV devices, however, several factors have to be considered. First, the exact location of the RA pacing lead may be relevant. Second, if prominent intra-atrial conduction delay occurs, LA activation can be delayed, and since with BiV systems, the LV lead is programmed to pace at the same time as the RV (or earlier), left ventricular stimulation may occur along with LV contraction simultaneously or earlier than LA contraction, producing left-sided pacemaker syndrome and often marked worsening of functional status.

The exact location of the atrial pacing lead may also be relevant because if the P-wave duration from that pacing site is long (deep in the appendage or RA free wall), then the effect explained previously (LA/LV dyssynchrony) will be exaggerated.

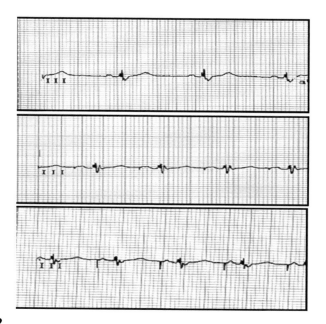

FIGURE 12

In Figure 12, the rhythm strip of EKG lead III is shown. Note that the P-wave morphology and duration vary in each of these panels. One panel shows sinus rhythm; another, RA pacing from the RA appendage; and another, pacing from the high interatrial septum (Bachmann bundle). Can you identify which rhythm strip corresponds to each of these stimulation locations (sinus, Bachmann bundle, and RA appendage)?

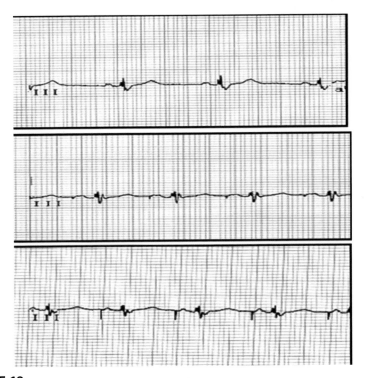

FIGURE 13

Figure 13 matches the stimulation site to the P-wave morphology seen in lead III. Each of these tracings was obtained from the same patient. Note that the P-wave duration is longest with RA appendage pacing, whereas it is relatively shorter when pacing from the Bachmann bundle. This is because of two reasons: first, Bachmann bundle has atrial myocardial fibers running parallel to each other on the roof of the atrium, facilitating RA/LA conduction, and second, because of the septal location of this pacing site, simultaneous RA and delay activation occur, and thus, there is quicker (narrower P wave) by global atrial stimulation.

If LA/LV synchrony is found to occur during BiV device implantation, the physician may purposely choose to place the atrial lead at a site that will "preexcite" the LA. However, this may not always be possible in diseased hearts, especially when an LV offset has been programmed. Thus, wherever the atrial lead has been placed in the RA, then LA/LV contraction may still be occurring near, simultaneously producing left-sided pacemaker syndrome.

In these instances (diseased atria and LV offset programmed on), ideally, the LA should be paced and the LA/LV time programmed accordingly. How can one pace the LA?

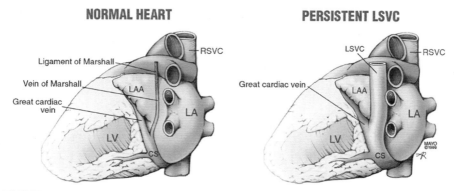

FIGURE 14

Figure 14 shows the anatomy of the left superior vena cava (right panel) and its remnant to the vein/ligament of Marshall. The vein of Marshall, when present, drains to the coronary sinus just as the left superior vena cava did in fetal life. Just as we pace the LV through the coronary venous system and the LV veins, the LA can be paced through the coronary venous system and its LA tributaries.

CASE SERIES 2

Case 2.1 Why Does the Morphology Change?

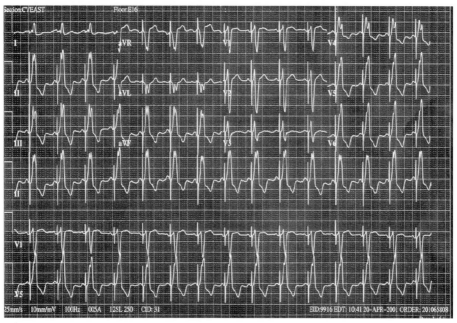

FIGURE 1 Biventricular pacing: left ventricular output, 5 V at 0.5 msec.

Figure 1 is a 12-lead electrocardiogram obtained from a patient with a biventricular (BiV) pacing device. Both right ventricular (RV) and left ventricular (LV) lead function was found to be normal, and the LV pacing threshold was 0.5 V at 0.5 msec.

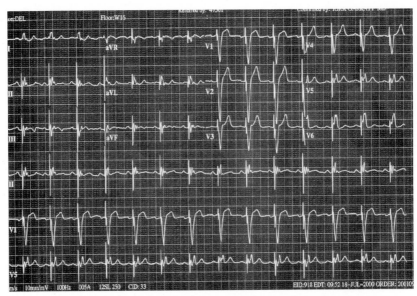

FIGURE 2 Biventricular pacing: left ventricular output, 1 V at 0.5 msec.

The electrocardiogram shown in Figure 2 was obtained in the same patient with no change in the location of the LV pacing lead and at a similar pacing rate. The only difference was in the programmed output. The reader will note that the programmed output was still well above the LV pacing threshold that had just been obtained.

Why is it that the paced morphology has changed so significantly between Figures 1 and 2?

    A) The left ventricular lead moves with respiration

    B) There is intermittent loss of capture in the left ventricular lead

    C) There is intermittent loss of capture on the right ventricular lead

    D) Anodal stimulation is present

    E) None of the above

Answer D: Anodal stimulation is present

Note specifically in the inferior leads (II, III, and aVF) with lower output pacing that the R-wave amplitude is greatly decreased. Also, lead aVL goes from being negative with high output pacing to positive with lower output pacing.

128

This phenomenon where the pacing vector can change significantly is termed *anodal stimulation*. The LV lead in this patient has been placed in an anterior location. With lower output pacing, there is anodal stimulation with relative greater contribution to ventricular stimulation from the RV lead, and thus, the expected tall R waves (LV anterior pacing) are not seen at lower output pacing. When anodal stimulation occurs, the benefit of the LV pacing lead is no longer possible (because the pacing wavefront emanates from the RV [anode]). If this is observed during electrocardiography in patients who are nonresponders to cardiac resynchronization therapy, changing the output appropriately may be beneficial.

Case 2.2   Capture with Delay

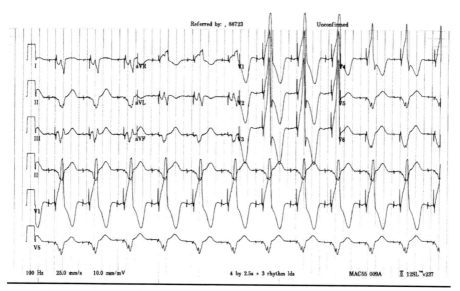

FIGURE 3   Left ventricle–only pacing.

The electrocardiogram shown in Figure 3 is from a patient with ischemic cardiomyopathy obtained during device testing. Note that with LV pacing, the expected right bundle branch block morphology is seen. However, when one looks at lead I or aVL (left-sided leads), the initial portion is isoelectric (slightly negative), and then after a prolonged delay, a short negative deflection results. This is consistent with prominent exit delay from the LV pacing site. Capture latency can also produce a similar phenomenon where the expected wavefront (away from lead I) occurs but does not do so immediately after the pacing spike.

Can you predict what biventricular pacing with no offset would look like in such a patient?

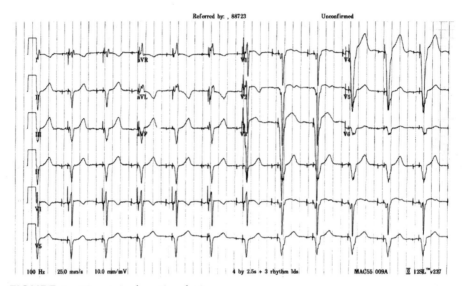

FIGURE 4 Biventricular stimulation.

Note that with BiV stimulation, an almost entirely RV wavefront is seen with left bundle branch block and an R wave in lead I and aVL. Note also, however, that the QRS duration is significantly less despite the RV pacing wavefront (60 msec less). QRS duration is a poor predictor of clinical outcome, and the RV pacing vectors suggest that the patient would have just as well with RV pacing alone. In fact, RV pacing and BiV stimulation electrocardiograms were nearly indistinguishable. BiV stimulation is shown in Figure 4.

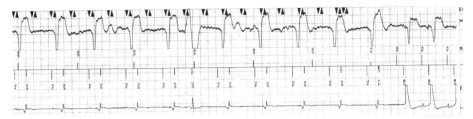

FIGURE 5

Capture latency, as well as prominent exit delay or interventricular conduction delay, can be seen during device interrogation as well. Note for example in Figure 5 that during LV amplitude threshold testing, LV pacing results in consistent capture; however, the RV lead (VS) senses the paced wavefront with prominent intraventricular conduction delay. This is an approximation of the interventricular (interlead) conduction time and can be used when optimizing devices to find the appropriate LV offset. Note the QRS morphology change in BiV stimulation seen at the *right* end of the tracing. Incidentally, in prior BiV implantable cardioverter defibrillator devices, this phenomenon could have given rise to double counting and inappropriate detection of ventricular arrhythmia.

CASE SERIES 3

Case 3.1 Troubleshooting Difficulty with Left Ventricular Lead Implantation

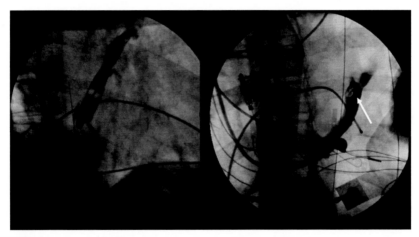

FIGURE 1

From Asirvatham S. Anatomy of the coronary sinus. In: Yu CM, Auricchio HD, eds. *Cardiac Resynchronization Therapy*. Oxford: Blackwell/Futura; 2006:211–238).

In Figure 1, the right anterior oblique (RAO; left panel) and left anterior oblique (LAO; right panel) views with coronary sinus (CS) angiography are shown prior to left ventricular (LV) lead implantation.

The patient had a previous attempt that failed; what is the likely cause or difficulty with left ventricular lead lateral wall placement in this patient?

A) Occlusion of the coronary sinus

B) Proximal coronary sinus dissection

C) Valve near the posterolateral vein

D) Prominent valve at the coronary sinus ostium

E) None of the above

Answer C: Valve near the posterolateral vein

This patient has valves in the coronary venous system. The arrow in the LAO projection points to an example of the Vieussen valve. This is a fairly consistent but usually small valve that guards the ostium of the posterolateral tributary of the CS. When present and large, as in this case, it can be difficult to advance a pacing lead to a venous tributary on the lateral wall.

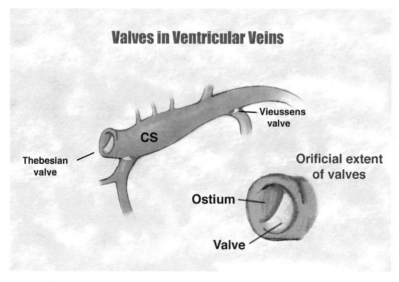

FIGURE 2

From Asirvatham S. Anatomy of the coronary sinus. In: Yu CM, Auricchio HD, eds. *Cardiac Resynchronization Therapy*. Oxford: Blackwell/Futura; 2006:211–238).

Valves may occur at several locations in the coronary venous system (Figure 2). The Thebesian valve guards the opening of the CS, and valves may also be found at the ostium of the middle cardiac vein. The orificial extent of these valves is highly variable, and they rarely can be nearly occlusive.

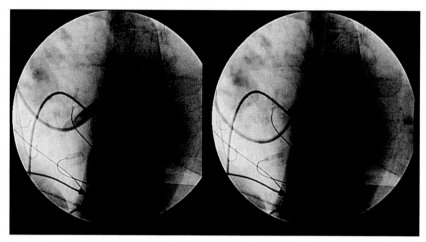

FIGURE 3

Another cause for difficulty in placing an LV lead is illustrated in Figure 3. In the left panel, an abrupt narrowing in the midportion of the CS (CS stenosis) is seen. Low-pressure and balloon dilation was performed, and the relatively normal distal vessels of the coronary venous system are seen in the right panel.

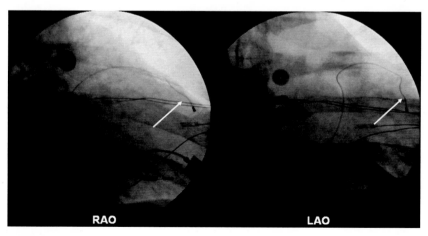

FIGURE 4

RAO and LAO projections of biventricular lead implantation are shown in Figure 4.

Can you make a prediction on how the electrocardiogram would look? Do you think this left ventricular pacing site will help the patient?

In the RAO projection, it is clearly evident that the LV lead (arrow) is clearly traversing the anterior interventricular vein. However, in the LAO projection, we note that the lateral tributary has been subselected. Thus, despite the fact that the anterior vein was used, a lateral site is where the pacing lead wound up and is being used for stimulation. This principle that tributaries of any of the major coronary venous systems can be cannulated to reach the lateral wall is important to keep in mind. Sometimes, the lateral vein may be atretic or have a stenotic segment or a large Vieussen valve, and in those cases, instead of considerable time and difficult manipulation to get into that vein, a tributary of the anterior vein will give just as good a result with less risk, and so on.

Case 3.2 Difficulties Continued

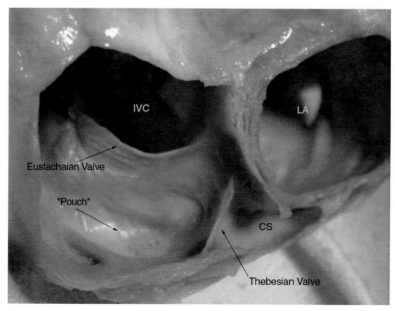

FIGURE 5

If a patient with planned left ventricular lead implantation were to have the anatomy shown in Figure 5, what would be the primary cause of difficulty in performing the procedure?

A) A large Thebesian vein is present and will not allow access to the CS.

B) A subeustachian pouch is present.

C) A large Eustachian ridge and valve will make it difficult to cannulate the coronary sinus.

D) There is no significant cause for difficulty and the procedure should go smoothly.

Answer B: A subeustachian pouch is present

Although large Thebesian valves can be problematic, they rarely are occlusive, and with the correct technique (starting with the guiding catheter sheath or wire from a ventricular location and then rotating into the CS while pulling back), it can usually easily be crossed. Subeustachian pouches, however (often associated with large Thebesian valves), can make CS cannulation exceedingly difficult. The reason for this is two-fold: (1) guiding catheters will be seated too deep into the pouch, and when a wire or lead is advanced from the guide catheter, it will tend to travel up the interatrial septum; and (2) when difficulty is noted while trying to enter the CS, operators often will puff contrast dye to see whether the CS ostium can be visualized.

In Figure 6, when the guide (through which the dye is being injected) is in a pouch, the contrast will tend to swirl and appear stagnant. If this is mistaken for a poor location, then the operator will continue to torque the sheath more posteriorly, and once the sheath falls behind the Eustachian ridge, the CS can never be cannulated from that location. Knowledge of the pouch and the fact that swirling contrast may suggest that the correct plane has been appropriate, change of sheath or manipulation can lead to successful CS cannulation.

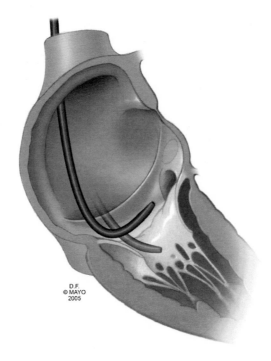

FIGURE 6

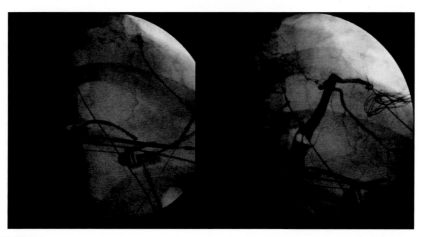

FIGURE 7

Another potential pitfall with angiography is shown in Figure 7. The right panel shows CS angiography, and there is no clearly apparent posterior or posterolateral vein that could be used for LV lead implantation. The left panel, however, illustrates that with a deflectable catheter, a relatively large posterolateral vein (subselection with a guide catheter has taken place fairly easily) that would be an excellent location for placing an LV lead has been found. Coronary angiography may yield misleading results when complete occlusion has not occurred or the balloon itself sits near the ostium of the vein, or the balloon has been placed too distally into the coronary sinus.

CASE SERIES 4

Case 4.1   Troubleshooting Failure to Improve— Electrocardiographic Correlation

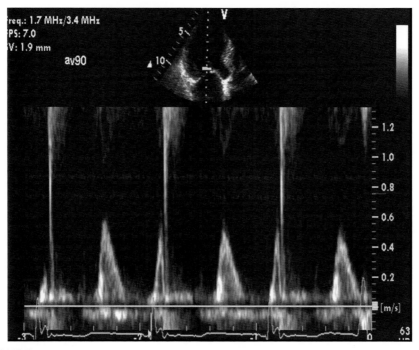

Freq.: 1.7 MHz/3.4 MHz
FPS: 7.0
V: 1.9 mm
av90

FIGURE 1

The mitral inflow Doppler tracings in a patient with a biventricular pacing device are shown in Figure 1. Would you predict benefit at these program settings (AV interval, 90 msec) for the patient? Can you identify the "E" (early filling) and "A" (atrial systole) waves on the mitral inflow Doppler?

The A wave is truncated; that is, mechanical ventricular systole has begun even before complete atrial emptying into the left ventricle (LV). This is the mechanical equivalent of left atrium (LA)–LV electrical dyssynchrony. Pulmonary capillary pressures may rise, and the patient paradoxically develops worse symptoms of congestive heart failure after device implantation when the AV interval is too short.

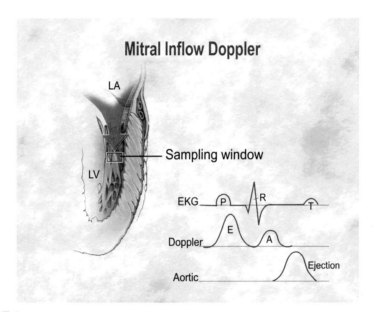

FIGURE 2

The principle of using mitral inflow Doppler to identify optimal LA-LV synchrony is illustrated in Figure 2. Note that the "A" mechanical wave seen on the Doppler occurs much after the surface P wave. This is a result of normally delayed activation to the LA and the atrial electromechanical coupling time. Similarly, however, LV ejection seen on the aortic Doppler occurs after the QRS complex because of the LV electromechanical coupling interval. Thus, LA filling is complete or nearly complete before LV ejection.

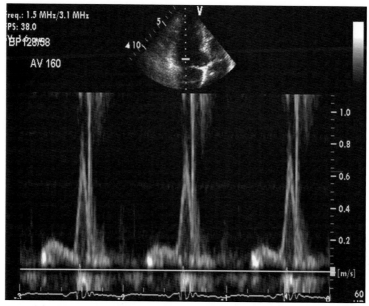

FIGURE 3

In Figure 3, the AV interval has been lengthened to 160 msec. Note that the A wave is now nearly completely seen.

Case 4.2 Programming Atrioventricular Interval

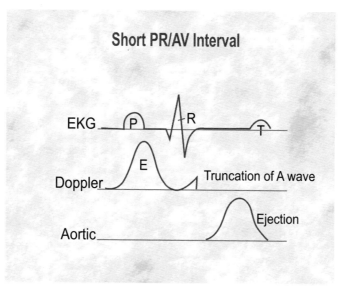

FIGURE 4

Figure 4 illustrates an extreme scenario where the AV interval is so short that the A wave is essentially not seen. This situation has been likened to atrial fibrillation; that is, the contribution of atrial systole has been removed. In fact, truncation of the A wave produces hemodynamics *worse* than atrial fibrillation. Because mechanical contraction of the atrium is occurring, except since the mitral valve is closed at that time, regurgitation through the pulmonary veins to the lung vasculature will be occurring.

With regard to programming the atrioventricular interval and resulting hemodynamic sequelae, which of the following is true?

A) An unnecessarily long programmed AV interval may give rise to systolic mitral regurgitation

B) An unnecessarily long programmed AV interval may give rise to diastolic mitral regurgitation

C) When the AV interval is programmed too short, diastolic tricuspid regurgitation occurs

D) When the AV interval is programmed too short, diastolic mitral regurgitation occurs

E) None of the above

Answer B: An unnecessarily long programmed AV interval may give rise to diastolic mitral regurgitation

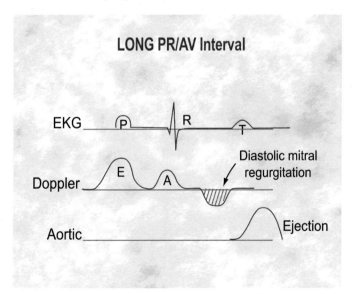

FIGURE 5

In Figure 5, the opposite problem of having a too long AV interval is illustrated. The A wave has clearly completed; however, because LV systole has still not occurred (long programmed AV interval), diastolic mitral regurgitation may occur and produce pulmonary edema or worsening heart failure symptoms. The optimal AV interval will be one in which the A wave is complete but there is no diastolic mitral regurgitation.

CASE SERIES 5

TEACHING POINTS

- Cardiac resynchronization: handling complexity
- Cardiac resynchronization: not responding
- Epicardial pacing
- Varying QRS width and morphology

Case 5.1 Cardiac Resynchronization—Handling Complexity

This case series will likely be of more interest to the advanced reader already familiar with basic biventricular device implantation and troubleshooting.

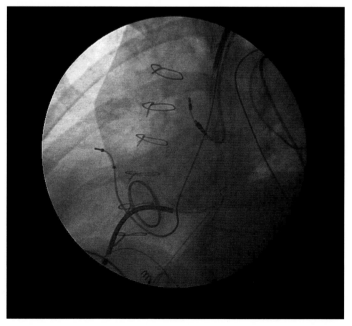

FIGURE 1

Case 5.2 Handling Complexity

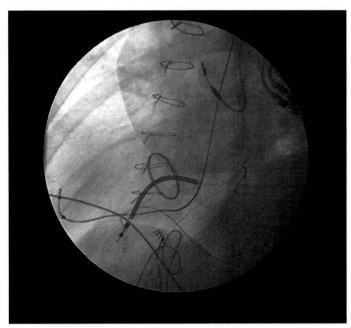

FIGURE 2

Figures 1 and 2 are two different pacing locations of the left ventricular (LV) lead in a patient with heart failure. After careful study of these fluoroscopic images, what are some of the challenges with LV lead implantation in this patient that can be identified?

What do you guess would be the main reason that the position obtained in Figure 1 was abandoned and the lead positioned as shown in Figure 2?

The first important observation is that both of these images (Figures 1 and 2) are left anterior oblique images (note the spine to our right). All pacing leads (atrial, right ventricular [RV], implantable cardioverter defibrillator, and LV leads) appear to be going the wrong way (to the right). This patient had congenitally corrected transposition of the Great Vessels along with dextroversion, with the apex of the heart pulled to the right. This is the first challenge that needed to be overcome. With situs inversus or complete dextrocardia, simply transposing the camera views (using the left anterior oblique as a right anterior oblique, etc) will generally orient the operator and the procedure continued. With dextroversion, the implant can be a little more difficult because of the portion of twisting that occurs to the cardiac chambers when the apex alone goes to the right side of the body. Second, an atrial ventricular valve annuloplasty ring is seen in both images. Patients who have had prior AV valve surgery may have challenging implants depending on how the valve ring was oversewn and the degree of asymmetric cardiac chamber enlargement.

Why was the left ventricular pacing site in Figure 1 abandoned?

Once you make the corrections in your mind based on the congenital disease, and so on, you would note that a high anterolateral location fairly close to the base has been obtained in Figure 1. Phrenic nerve stimulation or oversensing of atrial activity or capture of the atrium and poor thresholds may all be occurring in that location.

The lead has been moved using likely a posterior vein, and a tributary to come up to the anterolateral apex of the LV (Figure 2) was done with good pacing thresholds and an appropriate pacing vector.

Case 5.3　Still Not Responding

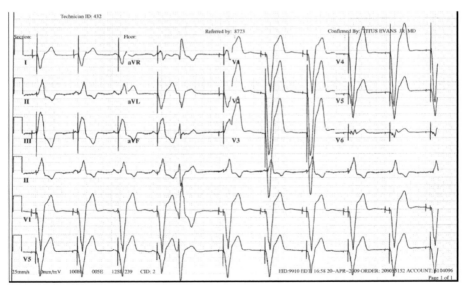

FIGURE 3

The electrocardiogram (EKG) during AV sequential BiV pacing from a patient who was a cardiac resynchronization therapy (CRT) nonresponder is shown in Figure 3. The RV implantable cardioverter defibrillator lead has been placed in the RV apex. Where is the likely location of the LV pacing lead? Could this location be contributing to the failure to benefit from CRT?

Although lead I is negative, suggesting LV free wall activation, the inferior leads are all strongly positive (R waves) in leads II, III, and aVF. There is also a left bundle branch block morphology. The likely LV pacing site is on the anterior wall of the LV. In this location, the primary vector goes from the RV toward the LV (left bundle branch block morphology) and in most patients is not an ideal location.

Can the reader predict what the fluoroscopic images would look like?

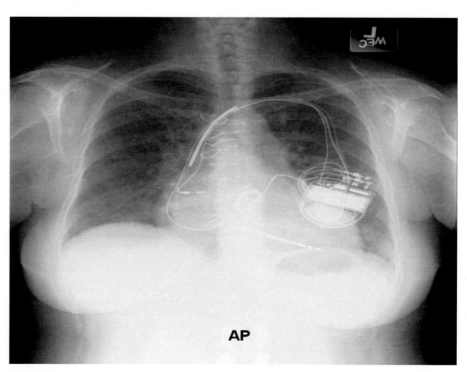

FIGURE 4

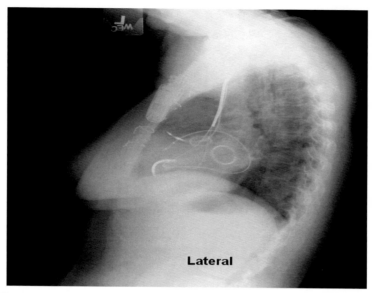

FIGURE 5

The anteroposterior (AP) and lateral fluoroscopic views from this patient is shown in Figures 4 and 5. Note in the lateral view that the very anterior location of the LV pacing lead is seen.

Case 5.4   Epicardial Pacing

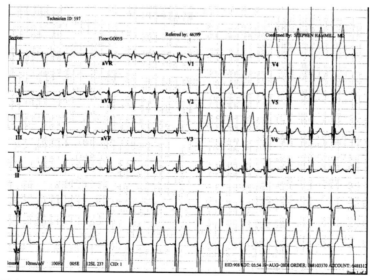

FIGURE 6

This EKG (Figure 6) was obtained in a patient with a surgically placed epicardial system. The QRS is narrow, and a QS pattern is seen in lead I. Note, however, the left bundle branch block morphology and strong inferior access very similar to what was seen in Figure 3. Epicardial implantation, especially if adhesions had been found by the surgeon and inadequate exposure of the posterior wall of the LV had occurred, winds up pacing the anterior even with epicardial implantation. Attention should be paid to the pacing vector. Appropriate optimization of lead position, as well as LV-RV offsets, when applicable, should be done.

Case 5.5   Varying QRS Width and Morphology

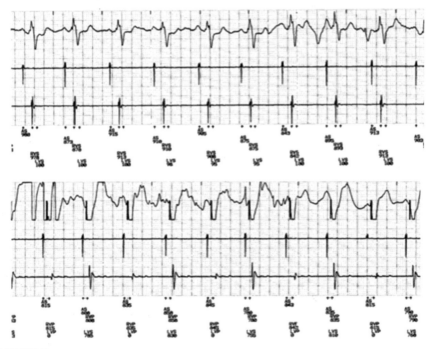

FIGURE 7

Figure 7 shows the retrieved data on interrogation of a BiV pacing system in a patient who had suboptimal benefit with CRT. Variation of the QRS during pacing at a constant output had been noted on surface EKG. The top panel shows the underlying rhythm, and the bottom panel shows data during BiV pacing above established thresholds. In each panel, the top line is the surface EKG, the middle line is the atrial electrograms, and the bottom line is the ventricular electrograms; the marker channels are also displayed.

What is the cause for the QRS width and morphology variation seen during biventricular stimulation? How do you explain the marker channel data?

In the underlying rhythm, sinus with intrinsic conduction is shown. There is a difference in timing of about 90 to 100 msec between RV sensing and LV sensing. This is consistent with left bundle branch block and LV activation occurring after RV activation.

When BiV stimulation is turned on, however, we note from analyzing the electrograms that there is an alternation in the height of the near-field ventricular electrogram. Corresponding to this, on a marker channel, we note that in every other beat, the LV lead does not pace, but rather, an LV sensed event occurs. The AV interval, when LV sensed beats occur, is also shorter. Although there are several possible reasons for this pattern, the alternation is likely a result of penetration from one paced beat into the fascicular system and myocardium of the contralateral ventricle. When this occurs, various manifestations of complex interventricular conduction and fascicular conduction in diseased hearts (cardiomyopathy existing bundle branch block) may occur and cannot entirely be predicted based on lead placement, and others. Furthermore, these changes may be dynamic (occurring during exercise, over time, as a result of added membrane active arrhythmic therapy, etc). The cardiologist caring for the heart failure patient with a CRT device must be alert to the various possibilities as to why a patient's clinical status may be worsening and be able to analyze the clues afforded by the EKG, echocardiogram, and device interrogation.

CASE 6 Analysis of Tracings during Device Interrogation in a Patient with a Biventricular Implantable Cardioverter Defibrillator

TEACHING POINTS	
• Ventricular sensing and capture • Latency	• Arrhythmia sensing • Threshold testing

Case Presentation

The following tracing was obtained during threshold testing of a biventricular (BiV) implantable cardioverter defibrillator (Medtronic Concerto).

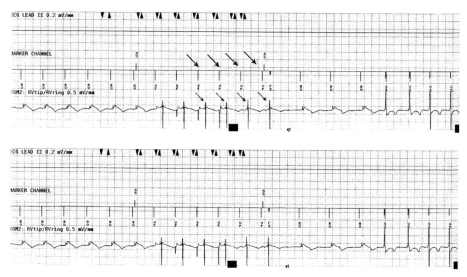

FIGURE 1 Top row: marker channels. Bottom row: right ventricular (RV) tip/RV ring electrogram.

Case Discussion

What observation can be made?

The first six beats demonstrate BiV pacing. The corresponding electrograms show capture of the near-field RV electrogram. The seventh beat demonstrates the onset of LV pacing (Vp). There appears to be two corresponding RV electrograms: one at the time of Vp and another exactly 200 msec (one large box) later. As the LV amplitude output decrements in the course of the testing, the first signal on the electrogram channels disappears (note no more signals after the fifth Vp). After this fifth Vp, however, and exactly 200 msec later, one can see another deflection, identical to deflections coupled with the previous four Vps. The sixth Vp demonstrates a similar finding, except in this case, the marker channel shows a corresponding FS ("fib sense") at the time of the RV deflection.

Although it may initially appear that there is no RV capture on the last two Vp beats, this is not the case. There is a marked interventricular conduction delay between Vp and RV sensing (so-called latency). The first of the two deflections of the RV channel associated with each of the first four Vp beats is far-field sensing of the paced LV impulse. The second is the actual sensed RV impulse. With the decrement in LV amplitude, the far-field signal disappears during the fifth and sixth Vp beats, but the RV electrogram does not. This is supported by the fact that what would have been the second of two signals coupled with each Vp continues at exactly the same interval as the Vp intervals (arrows). This suggests that the signals are causally related to the Vp. Thus, this suggests that LV capture must have occurred for the last two Vp beats, or else there would be corresponding RV activity exactly 200 msec later.

This level of conduction delay is quite severe and is not typically expected to be seen in normal hearts. Because the substrate in most patients who receive cardiac resynchronization therapy includes severe structural heart disease, this phenomenon is not uncommonly seen in patients with BiV pacemakers or defibrillators.

One final point: FS ("fib sense") can be seen after the last Vp. The reason is that threshold testing has ended, and now, the marker channel assumes sensing mode based on the RV signals.

CASE 7 Fusion and Pseudofusion

TEACHING POINTS

- Fusion
- Pseudofusion
- Biventricular pacing
- Failure to capture

Case Presentation

What observations can be made from the following rhythm strip?

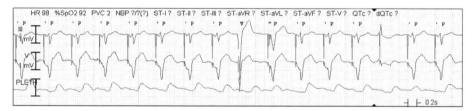

FIGURE 1

Case Discussion

The rhythm strip shows ventricular pacing and capture at a regular interval. The QRS width is relatively narrow, and lead III is not exclusively negative. These observations, combined with the obvious dual spikes, favor biventricular pacing. Thus, it appears that a device with regular biventricular pacing is operative. No atrial pacing is apparent, favoring either an atrial rhythm without clear-cut P waves or atrial fibrillation.

The ninth beat demonstrates a QRS that is obviously different in morphology. This may represent a conducted beat from the atrium or a PVC. Regardless, the timing of the ventricular spikes is not affected. The spikes may or may not be contributing to any myocardial activation. If they are, fusion has occurred. If not, the term *pseudofusion* is operative.

Further inspection of the tracing is revealing. The 10th paced beat shows a QRS morphology in lead III that is still different than the paced and 9th beats. This may reflect another level of fusion. More revealing is the 14th QRS. In this case, another premature impulse occurs. Its morphology is unlike that of any of the previous QRS impulses. The pacing spike remains on time but is relatively later than those in the eighth or ninth QRS complexes. Furthermore, the morphology of the 8th complex seems to be a fusion of the paced and 14th impulse.

In fact, the 14th impulse is a pseudofused beat with minimal, if any, contribution from the paced wavefront. Lead V_1 shows clear initiation of the QRS complex before any pacing artifact. Although we cannot be certain that pacing did not contribute to any myocardial depolarization, it appears to be to a less extent than the eighth or certainly the ninth impulse.

One final point: Let us assume that we had not seen a pacing spike in front of the fused or pseudofused beats. In this case, the variability in these (fused or pseudofused) impulses argues against supraventricular capture. If ventricular activation were to have been exclusively from a conducted atrial impulse, then the morphologies would have been identical.

CASE 8   Multiple Leads on Chest Radiography

Case Presentation

A 71-year-old man is referred for lead extraction due to implantable cardioverter defibrillator (ICD) infection.

You are presented with the following chest radiography.

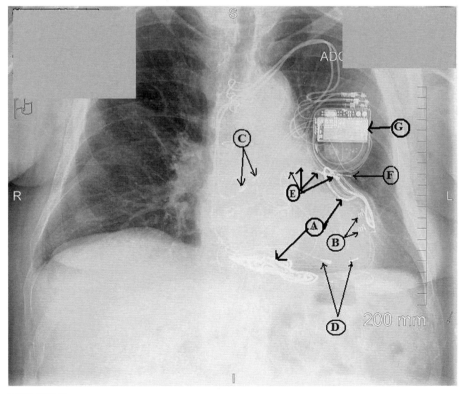

FIGURE 1

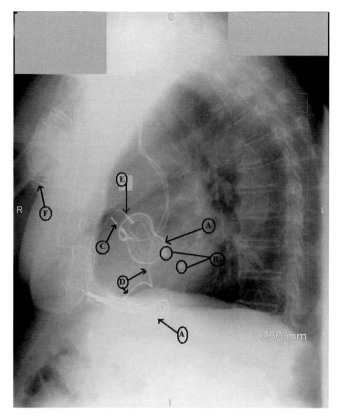

FIGURE 2

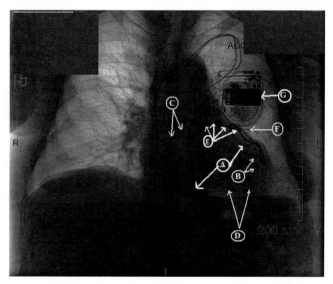

FIGURE 3

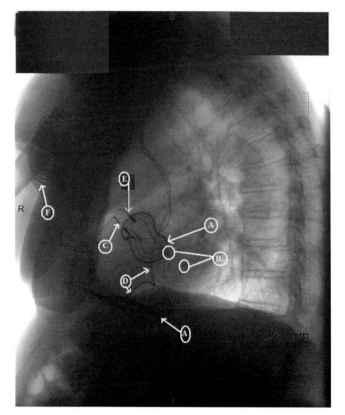

FIGURE 4

Case Discussion

Describe the patient's current leads/hardware

The patient has a left-side pulse generator. The size of the generator (G) combined with the presence of capacitors indicate this to be an ICD. Further confirmation that the device is an ICD is the presence of epicardial shocking patches (A). Epicardial patches were originally used for internal/implantable defibrillation. Epicardial pacing leads (B) can be appreciated. These are placed on the surface of the left ventricle (LV) (this is best appreciated on the lateral images as the left-sided structures appear more posterior). A right atrial endocardial pacing lead is appreciated in the atrial appendage (C). Note that on the lateral image, the lead is anterior relative to the left-sided structures and leads. The right atrial appendage is one of the most anterior cardiac structures. This is well appreciated on the lateral image. An endocardial right ventricular (RV) pacing lead is also noted (D).

Again, the lateral image is very helpful as it demonstrates the anterior location of this lead relative to the left-sided leads. In the lateral image, the lead traverses away (from the left subclavian vein toward the right atrium–superior vena cava junction) and toward the viewer in a forshortened manner (D) as it enters the right atrium, goes through the tricuspid valve, before finally coursing into the RV toward the apex. In the AP image, a pacing lead is noted to traverse superiorly. This may be entering the coronary sinus into a superior/lateral LV branch or it may be going into the RV outflow tract (E). Once again, the lateral image is revealing: the lead is anteriorly located and, thus, must be in the RV outflow tract (E).

Closer inspection of the AP image shows the tip of another lead (F). The location of this lead is better clarified on the lateral image, which shows it to be an old lead buried in the pocket (anterior to the sternum; F).

Leads in the coronary sinus (not present in this case; see images in the Biventricular Pacing chapter) will also demonstrate a posterior angulation, which is best appreciated in the lateral radiographic image (closer to the spine).

Some helpful hints: When confused about the orientation, remember that the spine is the most posterior structure and that the sternum is the most anterior structure. Sternal wires in patients who have had a previous sternotomy can be of particular help. Always order radiographies "overpenetrated" because this will allow more accurate demarcation of the lead tip. This is particularly important in patients with obesity.

Another tip is to use the features available on most computer-based radiology imaging stations. As an example of this, we have shown the original and "inverted" images of the same radiographic images for the patient described in the current case. Never underestimate the power of the lateral radiographic image. Whenever possible, this should be ordered. There have been anecdotes of patients with freshly implanted leads having lead dislodgement when they had to lift their arms for the lateral images. This is not an issue in a patient with chronic leads.

Because of the epicardial lead system, the patient required surgical and laser lead extractions. His LV function had normalized with LV epicardial pacing. Because he had had no ventricular tachycardia and was in chronic atrial fibrillation (developed after atrial lead placement), the only requirement was an LV pacing lead. All venous access was occluded, and thus, a second surgical procedure was required for epicardial LV lead placement.

FURTHER READING

ACC/AHA/NASPE 2002 Guideline Update for Implantation of Cardiac Pacemakers and Antiarrhythmia Devices (www.acc.org).

Baddour LM, Bettmann MA, Bolger AF, et al. Nonvalvular cardiovascular device-related infections. *Circulation* 2003;108:2015.

Baddour LM, Wilson WR. Infections of prosthetic valves and intravascular devices. In: Mandell GL, Bennett JE, Dolin R, eds. *Principles and Practice of Infectious Diseases*. 6th ed. Philadelphia, PA: Churchill Livingstone, 2005:1022.

Barold SS, Sinnaeve AF, Stroobandt RX. *Cardiac Pacemakers Step-by-Step: An Illustrated Guide*. John Wiley & Sons, 2003.

Buchet S, Blanc D, Humbert P, et al. Pacemaker dermatitis. *Contact Dermatitis* 1992;26:46-7.

Cacoub P, Leprince P, Nataf P, et al. Pacemaker infective endocarditis. *Am J Cardiol* 1998;82:480.

Chua JD, Wilkoff BL, Lee I, Juratli N, Longworth DL,Gordon SM. Diagnosis and management of infections, involving implantable electrophysiologic cardiac devices. *Ann Intern Med* 2000:133:604-8.

DiFilippo FP, Brunken RC. Do implanted pacemaker leads and ICD leads cause metal-related artifact in cardiac PET/CT? *J Nucl Med* 2005;46:436-43.

Eggimann P, Waldvogel F. Pacemaker and defibrillator infections. In: Waldvogel FA, Bisno AL, eds. *Infections Associated with Indwelling Medical Devices*. Washington, DC: American Society for Microbiology Press; 2000:247

Ellenbogen KA, Wilkoff BL, Kay GN, Lau CP. *Clinical Cardiac Pacing, Defibrillation and Resynchronization Therapy*. 3rd ed. Saunders; Philadelphia, PA, 2006.

Hayes DL, Friedman PA. *Cardiac Pacing, Defibrillation and Resynchronization: A Clinical Approach*. 2nd ed. Wiley-Blackwell, 2008. Hayes DL, Wang PJ, Asirvatham SJ. *Resynchronization and Defibrillation for Heart Failure: A Practical Approach*. Wiley-Blackwell; Hoboken, NJ 07030-5774, 2004.

Honari G, Ellis SG, Wilkoff BL, Aronica MA, Svensson LG, Taylor JS. Hypersensitivity reactions associated with endovascular devices. *Contact Dermatitis* 2008 Jul;59(1):7-22.

Uslan DZ, Sohail MR, St Sauver JL, et al. Permanent pacemaker and implantable cardioverter defibrillator infection: a population-based study. *Arch Intern Med* 2007;167:669.

Weiss R. Pacemaker dermatitis. *Contact Dermatitis* 1989;21:343-4.

Wilson W, Taubert KA, Gewitz M, et al. Prevention of infective endocarditis. Guidelines from the American Heart Association. A guideline from the American Heart Association Rheumatic Fever, Endocarditis, and Kawasaki Disease Committee, Council on Cardiovascular Disease in the Young, and the Council on Clinical Cardiology, Council on Cardiovascular Surgery and Anesthesia, and the Quality of Care and Outcomes Research Interdisciplinary Working Group. *Circulation* 2007;115. Published online April 19, 2007.

Index